Also by Townsend Hoopes

The Limits of Intervention, 1969
The Devil and John Foster Dulles, 1973

EYE POWER

Ann and Townsend Hoopes

EYE POWER

Improved self-awareness, vitality, and
mental efficiency through
visual training

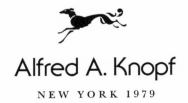

Alfred A. Knopf

NEW YORK 1979

THIS IS A BORZOI BOOK
PUBLISHED BY ALFRED A. KNOPF, INC.

Copyright © 1979 by Ann Hoopes and Townsend Hoopes
All rights reserved under International and Pan-American
Copyright Conventions. Published in the United States by
Alfred A. Knopf, Inc., New York, and simultaneously in
Canada by Random House of Canada Limited, Toronto.
Distributed by Random House, Inc., New York.

LIBRARY OF CONGRESS CATALOGING IN PUBLICATION DATA
Hoopes, Ann.
Eye power.
Includes index.
1. Orthoptics. 2. Vision. 3. Health. 4. Optometry.
I. Hoopes, Townsend   joint author. II. Title.
RE992.07H66 1979   617.7'05   79–2134
ISBN 0–394–50023–7

Manufactured in the United States of America
First Edition

To our children

Contents

Foreword

Ann and Townsend Hoopes have written the intelligent layman's guide to the new visual training. It is accurate, balanced, and interesting. It reflects a sound understanding of both the training itself and of the underlying scientific principles, and it is written in admirably clear and simple English.

Their book demonstrates, especially by reference to selected case histories, how the new visual training is helping to ameliorate or resolve a wide range of human deficiencies and discomforts that are related to vision and the eyes.

As experienced visual-training optometrists, we believe this book will be useful to everyone who suffers from a possibly correctable visual problem or from a bodily defect that is visually related. We hope it will be widely and profitably read by all persons who are interested in improving their self-awareness and the efficiency of their total performance.

Stanley A. Appelbaum, O.D.
Albert L. Shankman, O.D., F.A.A.O.
John W. Streff, O.D., F.A.A.O.

Introduction

This book seeks to report upon, describe, and explain a remarkable new approach to visual training, which aims not only at correcting defective vision but also—indeed primarily —at improving the general performance (meaning the physical, mental, and psychological efficiency) of the whole body/mind system. Developed and evolved by a small group of optometric pioneers, the program rests on the fundamental premise that vision is the dominant motor-sensory system, closely linked to the brain, and thus serves as the master coordinator of every part of the human organism. It follows that you cannot improve your eyesight, except very temporarily, without also improving your overall performance. In some cases it can favorably affect bodily ailments that are not generally thought to be visually related—though of course anyone suffering from such ailments should not defer medical diagnosis and treatment in favor of eye training alone.

This is a book for laymen by two recently convinced laymen. Both of us have undergone the training and have received significant, tangible benefits from it. From our own direct experience, we know it works. And the study we have made of its origins and evolution, through available written materials and extended discussion with a number of its leading practitioners, has confirmed and reinforced our own experience.

We have conferred extensively with Dr. Stanley A. Appelbaum of Bethesda, Maryland; Dr. Amiel Francke of Washington, D.C.; Dr. Lawrence W. Macdonald of Newton, Massachusetts; Dr. Albert L. Shankman of Norwalk, Connecticut; and Dr. John W. Streff of the Southern College of Optometry, Memphis, Tennessee. We have also interviewed and briefly observed the work of four other reputable training optometrists: Dr. Constantin Forkiotis of Fairfield, Connecticut; Dr. Israel Greenwald of Staten Island, New York; Dr. Sidney Slavin of Richmond, Virginia; and Dr. Bruce Wolff of Cincinnati, Ohio.

This book is intended to make more widely known the theory and practice of visual training, and what it can achieve. Primarily, we want to show people with visual difficulties or deficiencies how—if they are willing to make the effort—they can gain not only improved vision but also better health, better physical coordination, less stress, higher energy, and greater mental efficiency. The training program must begin with a diagnosis by a professional training optometrist, and must continue under his periodic supervision and assessment; it is too complicated and consequential to be a do-it-yourself program. At the same time, however, it demands the fullest, most active participation of the patient. Much of the training is done at home, and success depends heavily on a process of self-monitoring and self-correcting.

In our judgment, the program works because it is soundly grounded in a number of basic truths about the human organism that are now coming to fuller recognition and acceptance by science and medicine:

- that body and mind are interdependent parts of a body/mind system that functions as a unity;

- that the full and healthy functioning of the body/mind system rests upon the harmonious coordination of all its parts, especially the eyes, brain, hands, and feet;
- that good nutrition, regular exercise, and effective reduction of stress are the major ingredients of a longer, healthier, more energetic, more satisfying life;
- that the whole body/mind system, if we nurture rather than abuse it, can cure itself of most defects, and can also develop toward higher levels of mental and physical efficiency than most of us realize.

This last point is perhaps the most fundamental of all, for the old aphorism "The doctor treats, nature cures," to our way of thinking, sums up the entire scope and purpose of medicine. Doctors, whatever their specialty, seek primarily to provide sick or defective organisms with the internal and external conditions that will enhance their own self-regulative and restorative powers. Everyone understands that if there were no natural healing powers, medicine would be helpless.

Within the framework of these general truths about the nature of the body/mind system, a small but growing group of optometrists has over the past twenty-five years evolved a dramatic new concept of vision. Working in obscurity for many years, indeed faced with the indifference, skepticism, and even hostility of a majority of their optometric and ophthalmological colleagues, they have recently begun to find increasing respect and support for their views. The main reason for this acceptance is their dramatic success in helping children and adults to solve their problems in the real world: to overcome learning difficulties; to end frustration at being constantly tired, unable to read comfortably or to hit a tennis ball with accuracy; to convert failures in college and careers into quiet triumphs. One of the leading practitioners of visual training, Dr. John Streff of the Southern College of Optometry in Memphis, and a former associate of Dr. Arnold Gesell at Yale's Clinic of Child Development, believes the new approach is winning support because "it shows people they can gain a larger measure of control over their own lives. It is personal, individualistic, and it moves toward positive adaptations and enhancement. In this sense it compares very favorably to medicine, which increasingly treats with drugs and confronts the individual with large, impersonal bureaucratic organizations."

While we have tried to explain everything in simple English, we do provide a glossary at the back of the book to clarify the meaning of certain technical terms.

EYE POWER

One

What Is
Visual Training?

THE OPTOMETRISTS belonging to the new school of
visual training are strong individuals. They are also, however,
products of exposure to a common body of training doctrine
developed primarily by or within the Optometric Extension
Program, a nonprofit education and research foundation
located at Duncan, Oklahoma. While they differ slightly
from each other in matters of detail, they share a broad base
of proven procedures for exercising the eyes and for improving posture and enhancing bodily balance and coordination.
There is among them full agreement on the set of basic
propositions that define and distinguish the new school of
visual training. These propositions are that—

1. the eyes are not a camera simply recording what is
   objectively in the environment, but are receptors of the
   brain;

3

2. eyesight may be defined as merely seeing, but vision involves synthesizing, unifying, and understanding what is seen;
3. vision is therefore no mere passive event, but a complicated and largely a learned process that occurs mainly in the brain;
4. from birth, each person develops his own "space world," and that increasingly elaborate and subtle complex greatly influences the development of his thought patterns and his personality;
5. the building blocks of vision are the simple space/time relationships that exist between each person and the objects in his field of vision;
6. a person's ability to locate, interpret, and manipulate physical objects in his field of vision is directly related to his ability to deal with abstract concepts and ideas—that is, to his ability to think, create, and solve problems;
7. posture and vision interact;
8. many visual problems are caused or aggravated by postural distortions, and many ailments connected with posture (including backaches and pinched nerves) are caused or aggravated by defective vision;
9. stress, which affects the whole body/mind system, including specifically the visual system, drains away finite energy and constricts performance.

Optometrists who base their professional practice on these propositions are disciples, directly or indirectly, of a remarkable man, Dr. A. M. Skeffington, whom they regard as "the apostle of remedial visual care" and the single most important pioneer in the field of visual training. Born in Nebraska at the turn of the century, of a seafaring English father and an intellectual Danish mother who was educated at the "royal court school" in Copenhagen, Skeffington was a man strongly marked by an ascetic discipline, an insatiable curiosity, and a passion for logic. These qualities having apparently persuaded his parents and religious mentors that he was a natural for a career in the church, he was sent to a theological seminary at Nashota, Wisconsin, but quit within a year when he concluded that life as a clergyman would require him, as he put it, to abandon reason. According to his own account, he found secular education equally unsatisfactory and so he dropped out of school altogether and went West for several years to herd sheep, wrangle cattle, pick hay, and work on a railroad section gang. Eventually he drifted into the study of optometry. In that calling, he seems to have found the lifelong challenge to discipline, logic, and imagination he was seeking. Largely self-educated, he probed the mysteries of human vision with a monastic zeal, showing little interest in money, and indifference to food, clothing, and other material trappings. In the early 1920s he was the first educational director of the Optometric Extension Program, and for forty years thereafter the guiding spirit of this organization, which was and remains the principal focal point for those optometrists seeking to advance the cause of remedial visual training. He traveled widely and incessantly—one colleague called him "optometry's circuit rider"—to lecture and discuss, challenging the conventional wisdom of a conventional profession with a fine cutting edge and continually examining and reexamining his own positions.

Skeffington discovered and coherently explained a number of the propositions that now characterize and underpin the new school of visual training:

- In the 1920s, he showed that reading, or any near-centered visual task sustained over considerable stretches of time, is "an affront and insult to the natural and primitive use of eyesight," and that the eye's reaction is to go into myopia (nearsightedness).

- Also in the 1920s, he showed that the single test of distance vision (the familiar Snellen chart that tests the eyes at 20 feet in relation to what they should see at 20 feet) provides a seriously inadequate assessment of visual performance. He showed that large numbers of people who test 20/20 are nevertheless poor readers because their eyes do not focus well or coordinate with each other at short ranges. Eye tests arranged by Dr. Skeffington showed that most students in the bottom third of their elementary school classes possessed excellent distance vision, and similar tests today show the same results.

- From his conclusion that the Snellen test was inadequate, Dr. Skeffington developed an 18-point optometric examination, which later became the 21-point examination now certified by the Optometric Extension Program and used by all practitioners of the new school of visual training. This examination tests for eye muscle action, side vision, depth perception, focusing ability at near and far, and especially for coordination between the two eyes.

- In the 1950s, he introduced the notion that the *primary purpose of vision is to process information;* that is, to select items from among the millions of stimuli presented to the visual system, to identify these, to analyze and match them against the cumulative experience of the whole organism, to "see" them in a way that is conditioned by this synthesis with previous experience, and then to apply what is "seen" to the task at hand—whether it be finding your way to your seat in a darkened theater or trying to understand an esoteric poem.

• These and other of Dr. Skeffington's specific insights, when taken together, formed the basis for the radical theory that vision is in major respects a learned skill, as complex a process as learning to speak. Visual deficiencies should not therefore be regarded as fixed, irreversible physical flaws, but as correctable through training—proper training that can lead the whole body/mind system to see more efficiently, in the double sense of "seeing" and "understanding."

Those who followed and believed in Skeffington have of course built up and amplified his insights, adding valuable findings of their own through research, observation, and direct experience with their patients. Believing that the visual system leads, coordinates, and thus greatly influences all functions of the body/mind system, the new school optometrists have developed a comprehensive, holistic approach to visual training aimed at improving the overall efficiency of the whole person. Because their aim is a more harmonious, more efficient relationship between vision, posture, muscular coordination, and the working of the brain, they measure success not primarily by improvement in the clarity and sharpness of the eyesight, or by whether the patient is able at the end to throw away his glasses, but rather by a better general performance, physical and mental, with or without glasses.

CONTINUING CONTROVERSY

Despite the great distance it has come, especially in the last twenty years, and despite its growing success and public acceptance, this new approach remains controversial. The Optometric Extension Program is supported by perhaps 3600 optometrists out of a total of 20,000 in the United States, and probably no more than 100 conduct what deserves to be called serious visual training. A number of reasons are advanced for this state of affairs. Serious visual training takes time, study, and commitment, and many optometrists are unwilling to impose this required extra effort on either themselves or their patients; it is easier, and no less financially rewarding, merely to prescribe lenses that will correct the eyes to 20/20. There is also the factor of active resentment on the part of some ophthalmologists (doctors who treat eye problems such as glaucoma and cataracts) and pediatricians who sense that visual-training optometrists are encroaching on their professional turf; while difficult to measure, this appears to reinforce a natural caution. But it seems fair to say that the overriding reason why visual training is still the doctrine of an elite minority within optometry relates to the innate conservatism, the powerful force of habit, the sheer instinctive resistance to change that characterize most professional groups, including optometrists. Optometry today is involved in a debate between the old "structuralists" and the new "functionalists," and, as the following case history illustrates, it is a debate that has been going on for a long time.

In 1942, Aldous Huxley, that quite unmedical man of British letters, restored much of his own failing eyesight after orthodox opinion had written him off as a hopeless case. He did this with the help of guidance and exercises provided by Dr. W. A. Bates, whose theories of remedial training for eyes were rather revolutionary at the time but have since been largely superseded by later discoveries and developments. Most ophthalmologists and optometrists, Huxley wrote, consider eyes to be "totally different in kind from other parts of the body," from which they conclude that "defects in the organs of seeing are incurable and can only be palliated by the mechanical neutralization of symptoms"; accordingly, they believe it is "a waste of time even to try to discover a treatment which will assist nature in its normal task of healing"—the only "solution" is to fit the eyes with the permanent crutch of artificial lenses.

Huxley considered this a "radically wrong" approach, and he drew an analogy between eyes and other organs of the body. "Suppose that crippled eyes could be transformed into crippled legs. What a heart-rending parade we would witness on a busy street! Nearly every other person would go limping by. Many would be on crutches and some in wheelchairs." But, Huxley argued, when legs are crippled, doctors refuse to let their patients rely indefinitely on crutches; they regard crutches as merely a temporary expedient, and they apply their highest skills to improving the internal conditions of the defective part, so that nature can do its own work of healing. The measures they apply include rest, massage, applications of heat and light, and gradually increased exercise. Their purpose is to relax the defective part, increase its circulation, and preserve its mobility.

"If such things can be done for crippled legs," Huxley asked, "why should it not be possible to do something analogous for defective eyes?" To this question he found that "the orthodox theory provides no answer—merely takes it for granted that the defective eye is incurable and cannot, in spite of its peculiarly intimate relationship with the psyche, be reeducated toward normality by any process of mind/body coordination." The exasperated Huxley found such orthodoxy "so implausible, so intrinsically unlikely to be true, that one can only be astonished that it should be so generally and so unquestioningly accepted. Nevertheless, such is the force of habit and authority that we do all accept it."

OLD SCHOOL VS. NEW SCHOOL

While several significant scientific developments, especially the theory of the feedback process called cybernetics, have reinforced the new approach, the debate between "structuralists" of the old school and "functionalists" of the new is still very much alive. The conventional, old school optometrists regard vision as something that happens to a person with a minimum of self-involvement, and that accordingly bears little or no relationship to the person's general behavior, level of energy, state of health, bodily coordination, or worldly achievement. The optical systems are regarded as responding in a rather automatic, instinctive manner to light and light patterns. When this happens in an orderly manner, and where there is no eye damage or disease, the necessary conditions for satisfactory seeing are considered to be present. Practitioners of the new school, on the other hand, regard vision as an active process engaging both the brain and the nervous system, and operating at birth through a series of reflexes that are progressively modified and elaborated by the person's conscious response to experience; in their view, vision is, to a large degree, something that people learn to do.

Old school structuralists regard visual defects—"refractive errors"—as genetically predetermined and basically unchangeable; new school functionalists view such defects as at least potentially repairable. Both groups would agree that a patient with an acuity of 20/40 (on the Snellen test) can be brought immediately to 20/20 with the aid of corrective lenses. But, whereas the structuralist holds that the 20/20 acuity is obtainable only when the lenses are being worn, the functionalist believes that the patient can very probably be brought to an *unaided* 20/20 state through visual training.

The old school optometrist is basically convinced that the patient's only hope of improved vision is corrective lenses; his mandate is thus to "correct the refractive error" with spectacles or contact lenses. For him, the visual system can and should be treated more or less in isolation. By way of contrast, the new school functionalist sees "refractive error" not as a genetically determined, fixed condition, but as the surface result of multiple stresses or imbalances in the whole body/mind system caused by factors in the environment or in the person's lifestyle. Moreover, he believes such visual defects tend to develop in a predictable sequence and, unless corrected, become more and more deeply embedded in the structure and operation of the whole body/mind system. For example, the new school functionalist believes that sustained heavy reading will produce "near-point visual stress" which, in the absence of appropriate safeguards and countermeasures, will develop into myopia, or nearsightedness, involving a definite shrinkage and constriction of the range of visual performance.

Accordingly, while the functionalist is aiming for the same end result as the structuralist—to correct the refractive error in the eyes—he also seeks through training to *prevent* refractive error. In seeking to correct visual deficiencies, he believes that a number of other bodily subsystems must be modified, previously or simultaneously, because the components of the whole body/mind system are interdependent and interacting. While his basic belief is that vision leads and coordinates all of the other systems and subsystems, the functional approach to correction of defective vision involves more than eye therapy; it involves *simultaneous* efforts to enhance posture, balance, dexterity, and bodily rhythm. The functionalist believes that, through effective visual training including the appropriate use (for specific tasks) of stress-relieving lenses, the whole body/mind system will naturally reorganize itself in a more harmonious alignment. When this occurs, the obvious result will be not only enhanced visual performance but also more energy, better coordination, and greater mental efficiency.

Both the old and the new schools use lenses to assist in overcoming visual deficiencies, but they use them for different purposes and based on different assumptions, and it is important to understand these distinctions at the beginning of this book. Dr. John Streff has classified these lenses under three headings: compensatory, remedial, and developmental.

Compensatory lenses. The purpose of compensatory lenses is to make up for the refractive error in the patient's visual system, whether the trouble be nearsightedness (myopia), farsightedness (hyperopia), differences in lateral focusing power (astigmatism), two eyes that focus at significantly different distances (anisometropia), or cross-eye (strabismus). Compensatory lenses (whether set in conventional spectacles or contacts that fit directly on the eye) are usually worn all of the time, like a back brace or a crutch, for the patient cannot see satisfactorily without them; the assumption is that nothing practical can be done to *correct* the patient's underlying visual deficiency. Compensatory lenses do not correct, but merely compensate for. As might be expected, they are prescribed mainly by structural optometrists and ophthalmologists, for, except in rare cases, functionalists believe that deficiencies can be wholly or partially corrected, and they proceed on that belief.

Remedial lenses. These are also called *training lenses* and, as both names suggest, their purpose is to help bring about corrective changes and improvements in the eyes, or to help the whole body/mind system work toward better alignment and coordination. Training lenses are most often used when the eyes are poorly coordinated (they may focus at different distances) and when this inefficiency causes stress or bodily clumsiness. Training lenses are usually low-powered, designed to be worn for special activities (like reading or sports), and for relatively short periods of time. The lens prescriptions are changed after the patient's visual system has made an adjustment in the desired direction, and they are changed frequently as a means of pushing him further along the path to correction and better alignment. When the overall correction has been achieved, there is no further need for remedial lenses.

Developmental lenses. Developmental lenses are used almost exclusively with children, and for two purposes: to guide and reinforce visual development where the child has, through some accident or inadvertence, missed a step in the pattern of normal visual development, and to control the development of vision during the school years in an effort to prevent abnormal conditions—like myopia or strabismus.

For this reason, they are sometimes called *preventive lenses.* As structuralists do not believe the eyes are capable of change, they do not use lenses for developmental purposes. Dr. Streff argues for the use of developmental lenses by comparing our eyes with our hands and feet: we wear shoes to protect our feet from cold and hard pavements; when we play baseball, we wear a protective glove that makes it easier to catch the ball. Why, then, argues Dr. Streff, should we not give similar consideration to our children's visual systems, which are at least as precious and important?

Our purpose in writing this book is to explore and report upon—in terms understandable to the intelligent layman—what we have found to be a wonderful, workable approach to a healthier, more vital, more richly textured, more effective life. Visual training as conducted by leading practitioners of the new school is primarily for people with visual inefficiencies, or with mental and physical problems caused or aggravated by visual defects—and there are more of us in these two categories than might be perceived at first glance. *But amazing as it may sound, the program is also a proven vehicle for the enhancement, the self-improvement of those who are already performing at what the world regards as rather high levels of efficiency and accomplishment.*

Two

Personal Testimonies

A DIRECT WAY to show how visual training works is to describe our own family experiences with it. Ann's case is the most dramatic. Let her tell her story.

Ann Hoopes

In 1971, I contracted serum hepatitis from a blood transfusion given me during a hysterectomy operation, and the hepatitis subsequently produced a near-total collapse of my health. Cumulative stress had worn away my vitality and I had no more stamina. A number of bodily defects I had previously coped with now seemed to worsen all at once and to reinforce each other, so that I was very nearly overwhelmed. For the next three years I struggled arduously to get my strength back, with major help from a splendid nutritionist, the late Dr.

Francis Woidich, who prescribed no drugs but only diet and vitamins. He put me on a diet consisting chiefly of fresh fruit and vegetables, grain cereal, skim milk and yogurt, supplemented by large doses of vitamins, with emphasis on A, B, C, E, plus liver, calcium, magnesium, and potassium. I made steady progress toward recovery. Nevertheless, my body still suffered from numerous ailments and was generally vulnerable to viruses, bacterial infections, and other unpleasant visitations.

To list my major ailments is boring, but important in order to provide a reference point for the dramatic improvements that were later realized:

- One leg was slightly longer than the other, giving me an uncomfortable hip and back problem, more or less chronic and requiring continuous massage therapy for reasonable comfort.
- My natural posture was characterized by a slight forward tilt and a very flat back, which seemed to produce chronic upper neck and shoulder discomfort.
- My jaw frequently slipped out of alignment, causing discomfort and clogging one ear when I swam.
- My stomach was nervous and spastic; I suffered chronic headaches and inner tension for no rational reasons and contrary to my own belief that I was a calm, easygoing person.
- I suffered from the curious feeling that previous bouts of surgery had wiped out a good deal of my vocabulary; often I would lose a word in the middle of a sentence and grope desperately for a substitute, realizing even when I found it that it was not the precise word I wanted (I suspected this loss had been caused by the anesthetics given me in various operations).

Although I was making steady progress, Dr. Woidich was convinced that, like a number of his patients, I was losing energy through eyestrain, thus dissipating his own efforts to rebuild my bodily strength. It was true that my energy was still limited, but the idea that I was "losing energy through my eyes" seemed bizarre to me. I had worn spectacles since the age of 10, but had never thought much about it except that they were a nuisance and an embarrassment. Still, I was aware of my increasing need for them.

At Dr. Woidich's suggestion, I went to see Dr. Amiel Francke in April 1975. He examined my eyes carefully, then proceeded to tell me in terms I could understand why I did not see well: my eyes did not coordinate one with the other; I was nearsighted (20/100); both eyes were astigmatic; I suppressed one eye most of the time; my peripheral vision was weak. When I described to him my various physical ailments, he said they were, in some large part, the consequence of my defective vision, and he thought that visual training could help to correct them, especially my postural problems. I was skeptical, but I was also (at age 42) deeply depressed and frustrated by an accumulation of health problems that were debilitating, uncomfortable, and apparently insurmountable. Still I could not readily understand how eye exercises could change my body for the better. Dr. Francke said this skepticism was not unusual. He explained the interdependence of vision and posture, and invited me to come to one of his classes and talk to his patients to get an idea of what went on. So I began the training.

He told me the training would tend to add some stress to my already fragile system, and that therefore I would need more sleep than usual. Concurrently he would want me to undertake a program of physical conditioning, with emphasis on walking, jogging, swimming, and calisthenics to build up

17

the cardiovascular system in order to provide a protective cushion against what he ominously called "transitions." I learned that a "transition" in visual training is essentially a change from one condition to another—sometimes it involves an actual, slight shifting of muscles or blood vessels in your neck and upper back, signaling the realignment of your posture with your eyes; at other times it may be an awareness that your hand-eye coordination has improved. Sometimes, though not necessarily and not always, a transition is accompanied by temporary physical discomfort.

Each training class lasts an hour. When I began in May 1975, my limited energy allowed me to work for only about thirty minutes. I did three exercises: walking on an eight-foot balancing rail (four inches off the ground) while wearing (in rotation) four different pairs of "push-pull" glasses; tracking with one eye a small steel ball on the end of a wand that I moved in random patterns; and doing a "divergence-convergence" exercise with a stick while wearing "doubling glasses," which cause you to see two of everything. I later learned that these exercises were designed to "disorganize" or shake me out of my bad visual-postural pattern, as a prelude to developing one that reflected more harmonious eye-mind-body relationships. I also began my physical conditioning regime. Remarkably, I began to see and feel changes within a week. First, I had strange sensations in my neck and head—mainly a tingling feeling. Then I noticed that I could clearly see objects farther down the street and that the world was brighter. Dr. Francke prescribed new glasses for reading and a different pair for driving and distance, and he urged me to stop using sunglasses, on which I had depended for years; they were, he said, unnecessary crutches that would keep my eyes overly sensitive to light. After these initial changes, I soon noticed that my old glasses were too strong.

Over the weekend of July 29, 1975, I suddenly felt very tired on Saturday. Through all of Saturday night I had the sensation that gears were shifting inside my head; I did not sleep well and awoke with a headache over my left eye, and when I tried to read there were blank spaces on the typed page. Sunday morning, noticing that my distance glasses made things look too bright, I took them off and went for a walk. Suddenly I had the sensation of being eight feet tall, surely the strangest experience I have ever undergone. I was afraid to look straight down at the sidewalk for fear I would topple over, and when I returned home the furniture in the house had shrunk to half its normal size. When I called Dr. Francke on the telephone he said, "Well, you're having a transition. Go out for another walk or stay home and sleep, but don't read, watch TV, or do anything else with your eyes. Walk to balance out your body with your new visual alignment, or go to sleep." I did both of these things. In twenty-four hours the "transition" was over, and I was seeing quite differently. Everything was now consistently brighter and clearer, more intense—the way the world looks in the sudden sunshine after a rain.

My eyes changed again in August, and the doctor prescribed my next weaker pair of distance glasses (my old glasses were now uncomfortable). In late September I experienced another "transition." During the night I felt my back and neck bones shifting—they ached slightly for several hours, although I was able to relieve this somewhat by doing an exercise that consists of lying face up without a pillow and pressing the chin into the breastbone. Also I was inordinately hungry, and went to the kitchen at 2 a.m. for scrambled eggs and many pieces of toast. Dr. Francke had explained that I should expect this, for when the body is undergoing a significant muscular/chemical change, it needs more protein than usual.

The discomfort was quite worth it. When I went to eye-training class the following day, I looked out the window and found that the streetlights actually popped out at me. Dr. Francke was pleased to say that, after forty-odd years, I was finally discovering the third dimension. He sent me out to walk around the block. I went, feeling as though I were putting my feet into three-dimensional space for the first time in my life. I was actually a part of the scene; before I had always viewed it from outside, as though it were a flatland. This was one of the really thrilling moments. I have learned that such new discoveries happen frequently in visual training, and that the patient tends to weep or laugh with exhilaration. Some experts call it "critical empathy"—a momentary emotional crisis when you suddenly realize you are seeing things in a new way. Your first reaction is elation. Then you wonder how you could have been locked up for so many years in your old restrictive way of seeing, and the elation may turn to sadness. But then you recover, knowing you have made a breakthrough to something higher and better, and that you can consolidate your new position.

Meanwhile, I was undergoing some interesting body changes. My jaw was comfortably settling into place, my ear did not clog when I went swimming, and my back was somehow realigned so that now I stood both straighter and more comfortably. The persistent back pain was gone and my legs were the same length; I began to notice other changes—my shoulder blades began to fill out, and so did my bosom. My osteopath said he thought my upper back was "quite different" from the year before and probably would give me much less trouble. One weekend I discovered I now had enough curvature and suppleness to sit up and touch my toes, an exercise I had never before been able to do.

Since the end of 1976, life has become a rather thrilling experience. For the first time in my life, I can comfortably drive a car, play tennis, or watch a movie without glasses. I wear plus 75 lenses for reading, but no other glasses, and I have more energy than ever before. I wear no sunglasses, and the sun feels good on my eyes. My astigmatisms are almost gone, I see more easily and with far less stress, and I know I have become a more relaxed and a happier person. I can now think and express myself more clearly than I have been able to do for some years.

Though I ended formal vision training in 1977, I have continued to do several home exercises, as well as walking, jogging, and other forms of physical conditioning. I am convinced that further improvement—meaning an even better, more finely tuned functioning of my whole body/mind system—is possible. This is very exciting. The prospect for even better bodily health (for super-health), for further growth in visual perception and mental efficiency, seems, at age 45, a very good one.

Encouraged by Ann's successful response to the training, we decided to expose several other members of our large, rather sprawling family. None of the rest of us had any serious visual defects of which we were aware, and both individually and collectively we regarded ourselves as an outrageously healthy group, well-adjusted, athletic, and reasonably accomplished. Yet it became apparent over the space of a few months that certain visual or postural blocks were in fact denying each of us the realization of his or her full potential. When we asked Dr. Francke if our rich collection of eye problems made us an unusual family, he assured us this was not the case. In his experience, no one has perfect eyes or a perfect visual-postural balance. Some, of course, are much better or worse than others, but everyone has some defects, and some improvement is possible in every case.

Townsend Hoopes

In my own case, a moderate nearsightedness (of which I was aware) was shown to be aggravated by a condition of vertical phoria in one eye (meaning a tendency for the eye to flip up rather than gaze levelly). This naturally created a discoordination of the two eyes and was the cause of a progressive eyestrain and some noticeable fatigue. There were also several "tilts" in my posture, reflecting adjustments made long ago to both the myopia and the vertical phoria. The doctor found that the combination of visual and postural flaws was creating a general tension that drained away a good deal of energy. After eight months of eye exercises twice a week, both at home and in the classroom, plus regular jogging, walking, and swimming, the myopia was moderately reduced in both eyes, and the vertical phoria was substantially reduced—by about 80 percent, in fact. My only awareness of these changes was a subjective feeling that life was easier—I could carry my reasonably heavy workload of business and writing with less strain, I could solve professional and personal problems with greater facility, I had more energy for creative and athletic pursuits. Life seemed more interesting.

Cecily

Our daughter Cecily, now in her early twenties, was a lovely child, but shy and slow to understand things. Although she tested normally in a wide variety of school tests, she seemed to lack an alert perception of the "connectedness" of things, the intangible but important relationships existing between objects, events, or people. She seemed to see each object or idea in isolation, and her retention of what she learned was limited. As a result, she was rather withdrawn, slept inordinately long hours, and moved through the world with a tentativeness that reflected her lack of self-confidence. By dint of painfully hard work, and at the cost of great stress and fatigue, she succeeded in graduating from high school.

In the summer of 1975, in that breathing space before college or a career, we took her to see Dr. Francke. After examining her, he said, "This poor child has badly coordinated eyes. It is as though she were watching two different TV shows simultaneously, one with each eye, and trying to make a single coherent interpretation. Many people with a similar problem solve it by suppressing one eye. Cecily has been taking in conflicting images and information. No wonder she has failed to arrange them in meaningful patterns." He felt that visual training could help, but that a major effort would be required.

There ensued a truly exhausting year devoted almost wholly to walking, running, classroom and home training, progressive lens adjustments, and uncomfortable "transitions." Cecily had a slumped posture, suffered tension cramps in her stomach, and was overweight. The exercises, which improved the coordination of her eyes, also induced corresponding changes in her posture. Involving actual shifts in the muscles and blood vessels of her neck and back (and later of her hips and legs), these changes produced severe fatigue and occasionally "wiped her out completely" for a day or two. But the improvement in the coordination of her eyes with each other, in the alignment of her eyes with her body, and in her overall performance was measurable month by painful month. By July 1977, a number of changes were unmistakable: she was not only more physically fit and slender but also more mentally alert to the world and more interested in what was going on in it. She was more confident and outgoing. Previously passive and dependent, she now had a dozen self-initiated plans and the energy and discipline to carry them through, including college a thousand miles away from home. She still has a long way to go, but a year of rigorous visual training has given her life a coherence and direction it previously lacked.

Tom

Our younger son, Tom, 16, had no apparent visual problems, but was small for his age and rather low on energy. The visual training, which he took for one year, definitely improved his bodily balance and coordination, and apparently unlocked tensions in his system that were blocking his growth, for he grew nearly six inches during that period. His energy level improved, as did his general level of mental alertness and efficiency. This was reflected in both his academic performance (which rose from C+ to B+) and his athletic performance (where his new confidence and precision were noted by his coaches and teammates in soccer and tennis).

Andrea

In the case of our young daughter, Andrea, 9, her trouble seemed unrelated to her eyes. She was sweet, but vague, with a tendency to mind other people's business because she couldn't concentrate on her own. She had difficulty in school because she failed to listen, and she had difficulty relating to other people; she was also a bit clumsy. Visual tests uncovered a condition of vertical phoria and poor coordination between the two eyes. After a few months of wearing low plus lenses for reading, and also walking regularly a mile each day wearing "rotating prisms" for posture and balance training, she has become an attentive, observant little girl with an admirable attention span in reading, painting, and studying piano. Her academic performance is up. She has learned to ride a bicycle, and has become a beautiful swimmer as well as an expert performer on the trampoline.

Briggs

In the case of our college-age son, Briggs, 20, his eyes were 20/20, but the tests also indicated that he suppresses one eye at short ranges, particularly at the normal reading distances, which means he has been reading with only one eye for most of his life. His college schedule has thus far prevented his entering upon a regular visual-training program, but he is now aware of the handicap he labors under and plans to begin as soon as this is practicable.

Our own family experience has convinced us that a program of visual training, soundly conceived and conducted, has something beneficial to offer everyone, literally almost everyone.

Three
Vision and Posture

POSTURE IS LIKE a watchtower supporting the twin searchlights of the eyes. If it is strong and straight, the searchlights can scan an arc of impressive depth and width; they can coordinate their work, for each stands in the same relationship to the erect base. But if the watchtower is tilted, then one searchlight must view a given target from a different angle and distance than the other; coordination will be difficult or impossible. And if the watchtower is not only tilted but also wobbly, the uncertainties involved in trying to coordinate the searchlights, or in trying to make a coherent interpretation of the situation presented by the disconnected objects they are illuminating, are greatly increased.

Dr. Charles Sherrington found that "posture is an act," consisting of a continuous series of interactions with gravity and other reference points in the environment surrounding the organism. Together they add up to a "dynamic balance" as the various parts of the body perform the daily functions and tasks of life. Posture is therefore not static, but plastic and malleable, definitely affected by objects and movements in the outer world. Because the way in which the body/mind system perceives these objects and movements will determine its postural response, it follows that vision plays a decisive role in the development and determination of posture. Conversely, posture influences vision. There is a definite interdependence.

Darrell Boyd Harmon of the University of Minnesota, a doctor of both optometry and philosophy, has argued that a primary function of the visual system is to provide the organism with an accurate sense of its "exact and enduring position in space," and that this depends on maintaining the "habitual relationships of the main coordinates in your field of vision." The "main coordinates" are, of course, the vertical, horizontal, and depth dimensions in your surroundings, so Harmon is saying that a stable and upright posture is required if you are to perceive these basic reference lines accurately. But if the eyes are defective, then the vertical, horizontal, and depth coordinates will be perceived in their normal relationship only when the body posture is in fact tilted or otherwise "warped."

The reverse is also true. Dr. Harmon, for example, made studies of several thousand schoolchildren in Texas who had developed visual difficulties between the third and sixth grades. The studies showed that many of the children with visual problems also suffered "postural deviations" well beyond normal tolerances, and that these deviations were the primary cause of the visual problems. What caused the postural deviations? Dr. Harmon found it was a combination of factors in the schoolroom environment, mainly glare from windows parallel to the desks, flat-top desks that were too low, and large areas of dark chalkboard on the front wall that were difficult to see. In efforts to reduce the glare, see the blackboard, and write on the badly designed desks, the students tilted their heads, thrust out their chins, leaned to one side, or hunched over. The results were postural distortions that began to produce eyestrain over a few months; in many cases they set in motion a progressive interaction between worsening posture and deteriorating vision.

Why do eye defects lead to postural distortions and vice versa? Because it is imperative for the two-eyed human organism to put its space world in reasonable binocular focus or "binocular fusion"—the condition in which both eyes achieve an identical, mutually reinforcing focus on the same object. If one eye is weaker than the other, we instinctively squint and strain and make the postural adjustments necessary to achieve an approximation of binocular fusion. Conversely, if environmental factors cause postural shifts away from the ideal, the eyes must undergo corresponding changes, for the shifts will have brought one eye slightly closer to or farther from the target than the other eye; binocular fusion must then be achieved from an altered, slightly skewed platform.

The interdependence of vision and posture, and the adaptive capacity of the whole body/mind system are demonstrated by a simple exercise called binocular occlusion, which training optometrists frequently use. You can use it to test yourself. In this exercise you tape the inner half of each lens of a pair of ordinary spectacles (alternatively, use a simple index card), thus blocking out all frontal sight and leaving you with only peripheral vision (see illustration). Choose any

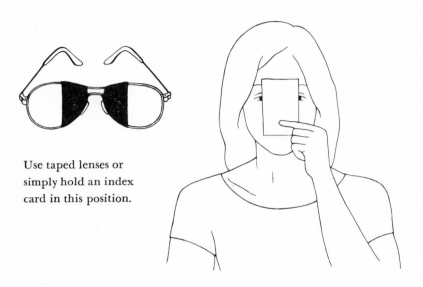

Use taped lenses or
simply hold an index
card in this position.

Binocular Occlusion Test

true horizontal line somewhere in the room—a shelf, door-sill, or table edge. Sitting or standing in a true vertical posture, you then look at that line, taking care to hold on to both left and right peripheries simultaneously. Being visually split by the blocking tape or index card, the line appears as two disconnected lines. If your eyes are equally good (or bad), the lines will meet if you mentally project them toward each other across the center gap. In the case of eight out of every ten persons, however, the lines (seen separately by the left and right eyes) will not meet if thus projected. In my own case (Townsend), one segment was slightly higher than the other, and one closer than the other. If that were the way each of us saw the world all day long, it would be an unsettling place, like a room of distorted mirrors in a fun house at the amusement park. We would orient ourselves only with great difficulty, and our anxiety would be increased by the knowledge, gained in earlier years, that such distortions do not reflect reality. To restore reality, we do a lot of adjusting, straining, and extra computing— which amounts to postural shifting. Some people "solve" the problem by unconsciously blocking out one eye. In my own case, I found I could eliminate the "binocular mismatch" by squinting hard and tilting my neck at about a 10-degree angle from vertical. It was a precise demonstration of the price in postural distortion I had been paying, no doubt for many years, in order to see the world more or less as it is.

The new school training optometrists have drawn from these studies, and from their direct experience with patients, the following conclusion: if you start with defective vision (no matter what its cause), you can assume that it will lead to some degree of postural distortion with accompanying stress, and may well result in a progressive inefficiency of your whole body and mind. Equally, if you start with postural distortion (no matter how caused), you can assume that it will adversely and perhaps progressively affect the visual system. It follows that, if you deal with visual difficulty and postural distortion as elements of a single problem, you can realize gradual improvement in both at the same time. This is the essence of the new school approach, and it explains in part why some of its practitioners place great emphasis on walking, balancing exercises, and calisthenics as an integral part of the visual-training program. These are the means to a strong erect posture.

A few case histories will serve to verify the interdependence of posture and vision.

Hans

Hans was a professional singer and musician who had been going to many doctors for years because his left eye was "quite different" from his right. He was aware that his two eyes didn't coordinate—the left eye wandered, leaving the right eye to do most of the work. No one had been able to help him. He wore glasses, but was uncomfortable whether he was wearing them or not. He was always tired, and suffered occasional double vision. Significantly, he suffered from a serious "postural warp," meaning in his case a severe tendency to lean toward his right side.

In optometric terms, the basic problem was a "high refractive difference" between the two eyes, meaning that the size of the received retinal image was much larger in the right eye than in the left. The approach to a solution was to put a contact lens on the left eye to reduce the disparity in size of the two retinal images and thus achieve a binocular focus. Then he was put on a program of home training exercises designed to improve his balance, coordination, and body awareness.

After three months, the severe rightward tilt had been reduced, and Hans's posture was generally improved. His back hurt from the shifts in his back and hip, but his three-dimensional vision was stronger. In addition, he felt he was singing more strongly, with more range at both ends of the scale; also, whereas he had always been a left-sided flutist, now he was ambidextrous. He was then given reading spectacles to wear over the contact lens on the left eye and the naked right eye, and these made it easier for him to read the musical scores while he was coaching and leading large singing groups. A year after his training began, the strength and muscle tone of his whole body were much improved and his nervous system was more relaxed. Although still thin, he had gained ten pounds. While there was as yet no significant improvement in his eyes (measured in purely optometric terms), he stood almost perfectly upright and felt that his vision was growing progressively stronger. In sum, the combination of physical conditioning exercises, balancing procedures, and specific eye exercises, plus the use of training lenses, had realigned Hans's body so as to make it more harmonious internally and more compatible with his visual defects. His whole organism was now better balanced and synchronized. He was "making relationships" more efficiently. The ground had been prepared for visual improvement in the next stage of his training.

Bethine

When Bethine began visual training, she was exceedingly tense and nervous, which the doctor discovered was caused mainly by contact lenses that were too strong—that is, they overcorrected her serious nearsightedness (20/250), making her eyesight sharper than her system could handle and creating physical stress. Her posture was typical of people who are myopic, or nearsighted—shoulders rounded inward, chin and lower portion of the pelvis thrust forward, the overall effect being a forward slump. The doctor prescribed spectacles with "a low amount of plus" to wear over the contact lenses, which had the effect of reducing the lens power overall. Then, over the next several months, he gradually reduced the power of the contact lenses themselves. Bethine faithfully performed a set of eye exercises under the doctor's supervision, as well as simpler home procedures, and she exercised regularly and adopted a high-protein diet. Eight months later, her eyes were 20/75, an almost fivefold improvement. Now she wears reading glasses over weaker contact lenses, but wears only the contacts for other activities.

The more remarkable change, however, was what the doctor called a "radical" postural shift, one that affected a bodily function apparently removed from the visual system, and with regard to which optometrists can claim no competence. She had a long history of menstrual difficulty and irregularity, and had twice been advised to have the problem corrected surgically, especially if she were contemplating having children. She rejected this advice and several years later undertook visual training without telling the optometrist of her menstrual problem. Three months after she started visual training, her menstrual irregularities ceased and she has menstruated normally ever since.

This is a case where a bodily malfunction was inadvertently corrected by visual training—where the combination of postural change and general reduction of tension resolved a serious condition of menstrual irregularity. The connection between the eyes and the pelvic organs, although apparently tenuous, was in fact close and direct.

IDEAL POSTURE

To Dr. Amiel Francke, "the level of efficiency of a patient's posture is a limiting factor on his visual performance, but postural changes should be gradually induced, just enough to support gradual change in visual performance." Dr. John Streff agrees with Dr. Francke and also emphasizes that, while posture and vision interact with each other, it is usually a change in visual performance that causes a corresponding postural change, rather than the other way around. Vision is the "lead system."

How do you achieve the ideal posture? The component elements are, of course, simple and well known to every physical education instructor: (1) pull your stomach in and lower your shoulders; (2) think of a tube running from your lower abdomenal region in the front to the top of your pelvic bone in the rear (it should rise from front to back at about a 30-degree angle); (3) tighten the muscles of your abdomen and buttocks to shorten the length of this imaginary tube from front to back and also to decrease its diameter; (4) make this whole effort without raising your shoulders and without producing excessive tension elsewhere in the body. In profile, the posture is correct if a vertical line can be extended from the midpoint of the ear downward to the top of the shoulder, the center of the hip bone, and the front center of the ankle. In full face, the vertical line should run straight down the middle of the body between the eyes, sternal notch, crotch, knees, and ankles (see illustration).

Why, it may be skeptically asked, does posture play a central role in the new visual training? After all, people with very poor posture manage to see. That is of course true, but the point is not whether they see, but how efficiently—how much straining, squinting, and postural twisting they must do in order to achieve a reasonable binocular fusion. The goal of a better posture is related to the broader goal of bringing about maximum harmony, economy, and efficiency throughout the whole body/mind system.

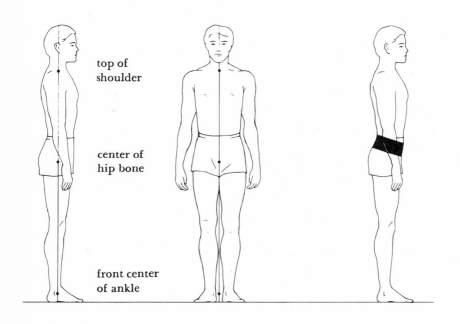

top of
shoulder

center of
hip bone

front center
of ankle

Ideal Posture

Efficiency is the name of the game. The person who is looking at a fixed object wants to know, indeed must know, what position his body occupies in relation to the object. He may wish to touch it or move toward it; he may want to avoid it if it poses a threat. But in every case it is necessary to his well-being that he correctly assess the angle, the distance, and the overall spatial relationship between the object and himself. The vital element in this assessment is vision itself, but posture is a determinant of vision. We cannot be well oriented unless we know where our head is in relation to the limbs with which we execute our decisive motor acts. Accurate grasps and precise motions with the hands and feet in relation to some visually fixed or moving object in space—whether it be a tree we are climbing or a tennis ball we are trying to hit—require coordination of the mind and eyes in the head with the arms and legs attached to the body.

The basic question is not whether a given task of brain-eye-hand or brain-eye-foot coordination can be accomplished, but how well and at what cost in physical and mental stress. Unfortunately, the efficiency and stress factors are usually ignored so long as the person under study is able to perform in an apparently normal way. The price of *apparent* normality may be in fact a tremendous amount of stress and inefficiency resulting in severe chronic fatigue and/or depression.

THE HIGH COST OF INEFFICIENCY

Dr. Leonard Cohen, in a paper on the mechanisms of perception, cited certain experiments with monkeys. After their normal ability to stand and climb had been tested and filmed with a motion-picture camera, the monkeys were divided into three groups and subjected to different kinds of surgery. In the first group, the vestibular apparatus (the semicircular canals and otolith structures in the ears, which provide our perception of upright balance) was removed; in the second group, the cervical components of the neck (which serve to orient the body to other objects in space) were removed; in the third group, both the vestibular and cervical components were removed. No damage was done to the motor system, to any other part of the brain, or to the spinal cord.

In the first two groups, general physical performance declined markedly for sixty days after surgery, then recovered to about half the normal level. In the third group, where both surgical procedures had been applied to the same monkey, the total deficit was much greater and recovery was less, but even here there was a significant recovery. Where the vestibular apparatus alone had been removed, the animals frequently fell over when they lacked some support to hold them upright. Where only the cervical component had been removed, the animals seemed to walk relatively well, but were notably inaccurate when reaching with their forepaws for objects on which they had fixed their eyes; for example, they showed great difficulty in climbing a ladder they had easily negotiated before surgery. Where both components had been removed, the animals had great difficulty both standing and grasping, *yet they managed to do both.*

What the experiment showed was that basic orientational components can be severely damaged without actually abolishing the body's ability to function, but that the cost in efficiency and physiological stress is undoubtedly very high. Bad posture similarly degrades *without actually abolishing* our ability to perceive the true vertical or to achieve tolerably good spatial orientation with objects in the space through which we move. But the necessary compensatory shifts in the pointing and focusing of our eyes cause tension, inefficiency, and loss of energy (sometimes in the eyes themselves, but also throughout the whole body/mind system) that is debilitating. It ought not to be ignored.

The remarkable resilience and adaptive capacity of the human body/mind system are well known, but the cost of major adjustment to unfavorable physical, mental, or environmental conditions is equally apparent. Instead of asking, "What extra drive can this person exert so that he can continue to perform adequately despite his deficient vision, poor posture, and bad coordination?" the new school training optometrists prefer to ask, "What changes can be made in the person himself or in his environment that will reduce the need for extraordinary exertion and will thus reduce the physiological stress?" In trying to answer the question in individual cases, they tend to believe that the potential for improvement in human performance is essentially open-ended. They note, for example, that, over the last twenty years, professional athletes have posted new records in a wide range of sports events, and scholars and researchers have continued to break dramatic new intellectual and scientific ground. Although the collective wisdom of mankind may seem at times inadequate to meet the challenges it faces in the fourth quarter of the twentieth century, the fact remains that individual human beings continue to advance to higher levels of both physical and intellectual ability.

BALANCED DEVELOPMENT

The new school training optometrists note that these ad-vances appear to be the result of *balanced* development, reflecting a higher coordination and efficiency between the major components of the human body/mind system rather than the perfection of any single subsystem. In this view they are supported by Dr. Arnold Gesell of Yale, who found that nature, through evolution, did not seem to be aiming at a perfect eye, but rather at a "plastic seeing mechanism," which can change as necessary to synchronize with advancements in the brain, hands, and feet, in order to permit an ever higher, more efficient action system.

This principle, advanced by Dr. Gesell, that balanced

development, rather than the perfection of any one organ, is the key to higher performance, may be seen in random examples of evolution. The eyes of a typical fish are set in the side of its head, giving it a narrow binocular field. Having no neck, it must turn its whole body to keep the object of interest within the range of both eyes. Now, a fish in water does not really need a neck, but when a fish aspires to a higher level of development—that is, to a life on land—the absence of a neck is a serious disadvantage (though not a greater handicap than the absence of hands and feet). Dr. Gesell cited the mud skipper fish as an interesting inter-mediate creature who couldn't make the transition, even though it had solved the eye-neck problem. The eyes of the mud skipper were set in high turrets on top of the head, giving it an enviable scanning arc of nearly 360 degrees. This seemed an ideal ocular adaptation to the requirements of terrestrial life. But the large pectoral fins, designed to pro-vide locomotion on the mud flats, were crude and clumsy paddle-like structures and were so poorly coordinated with the eyes that the mud skipper could not survive as a terrestrial organism.

Two factors were crucial to the higher development of the human eye and the human brain: one was the location of the eyes in a frontal position on the head; the other was the sophisticated development of the human arm and hand. For many creatures the snout, tongue, and teeth are the vital organs of prehension: the pig pushes, grasps, and handles with its projecting muzzle; touch, smell, and hearing are in his case of greater value than vision, and the visual sense seems to be quite undeveloped. Vision cannot become fully developed and versatile until the forelimbs are able both to sense and to manipulate, allowing the organism to guide and also to follow the movement of the forelimbs with frontally placed eyes. The relative immobility of the human eyes is more than compensated for by the extraordinary mobility of the head, which swivels on the neck. It is the coordination of the eyes and brain (the visual system) with the dexterous forelimbs that gives man his unique capability. This is seen, of course, in the work of skilled artisans (bricklayers, basket weavers), of the higher artisans (painters, sculptors), of athletes (tennis, basketball, lacrosse, and hockey players), but equally in the thoughts of thinkers and in every ordinary movement of the day's occupation. By progressive stages in evolution, the hand became more sophisticated and agile, because the eyes took note of what it was doing or where it was pointing, transmitted these observations to the brain, and the brain then sent new and refined instructions to the hand.

Nor is it possible to ignore the equally vital role of the feet, for they provide the essential platform for the postural set that gives man his distinctive skills. Dr. Gesell wrote that man's achievement of upright posture was the foundation of "new conquests in the sphere of vision," for such conquests require "a continuously harmonious adjustment between eyes, hands and feet." To return to our metaphor of posture as the watchtower supporting the twin searchlights of the eyes, the feet are obviously the base plates upon which the tower rests. Whether the watchtower is erect and stable or tilted and wobbly will depend on the strength and stability of the feet. Recognizing this vital point, some visual-training optometrists place special emphasis on walking as a conditioning and balancing exercise. A few put emphasis on the importance of wearing shoes that are wide enough to ensure that the ball of the foot is not cramped and that the toes are straight. In this view, shoes should be wide and relatively flat, for feet squeezed into fashionably narrow shoes cannot establish that solid platform for the body which is the foundation of good balance and posture. The result of shoes too narrow or heels too high is usually a tilted or unsteady walking habit that leads to bad posture and adversely affects visual perception. We will return to this subject in the discussion of physical conditioning in chapter 9.

Four

Vision and the Brain

EYESIGHT, AS WE noted in chapter 1, may be defined as seeing, whereas vision involves synthesizing and understanding what is seen. The visual system accordingly comprises not the eyes alone but also the brain. As Dr. Gesell wrote in 1949, the whole "human action system" is "governed by the input and output arrangements of the retina and the brain." Each eye, he said, transmits as much information to the brain as all of the other sense organs combined, for the seeing eye "is the most direct corridor to the vast network of the brain cortex, where billions of neutrons organize and engender the energies that issue in vision."

Dr. Darrell Boyd Harmon argued similarly in 1948 that a "purely optical theory of vision is inadequate"; it fails, Harmon said, to include the role of the brain in integrating experience and thus in influencing the way in which the eyes perceive and interpret objects and situations; nor can it explain the phenomenon of brain-eye-hand coordination in visually centered tasks (like writing and basket weaving), which involves a constant process of instruction, feedback, modified instruction, and control. The mere input of re-fracted light into the eyes, Harmon thought, has no meaning by itself; the eyes take in "something," but this becomes intelligible only when it is processed through the brain and the "body experience," where it is analyzed in relation to what the organism already knows from prior sight, smell, touch, taste, or intellectual experience. Dr. John Streff has explained this two-stage input-processing by reference to separate but intimately related motor and sensory systems in the eye and the connectors to the brain. The motor system, which is like a ready receiver, asks of a light stimulus, "What is it?" and the sensory system answers the question by iden-tifying the stimulus. Thus eyes and brain must work closely together to achieve coherent "vision"; otherwise, the result is merely an incoherent stimulation of the retina.

The new school training optometrists agree with Gesell and Harmon that the visual system embraces the eyes and the brain. They believe it is the "lead system" (to use Dr. Streff's phrase), the seat of command, the master coordinator for the whole body/mind system, receiving and synthesizing all the information supplied to it, integrating interpretation, order-ing particular limb and body movements, and organizing intellectual decisions. They believe vision thus plays a de-cisive role in how we move, coordinate, think, and solve problems—in short, in the development of judgment, char-acter, and personality. As Dr. Gesell put it, the visual system (eyes and cerebral cortex) is "a kind of meeting ground" where old experience is reconciled with new perceptions and both are assimilated in a new synthesis. It is where the "electrodynamic forces that culminate in adaptive behavior" —for example, the tendencies and skills required to become a research scientist, poet, business executive, or tennis player —are organized.

Accordingly, vision is not a simple, instantly realized function, but rather a skill that is learned slowly and cumulatively. Dr. Gesell wrote that the child "was born with a pair of eyes, but not with a visual world. He must build that world himself, and it is his private creation. . . . He possesses and refines it by a series of positive acts. . . . The space world thus becomes part of him. To no small degree, he is it." Moreover, the building of the individual's space world is a slow development over time involving the continuous interaction of eyes and brain, and thus a progressive expression of character and personality. Perception and response are both additive and cumulative, and it is this physical truth that gives structure to the learning process; all learning tends to utilize and build on earlier learning, instead of replacing it, so that most, and especially early, learning tends to be permanent; moreover, the more rapid learning capacity of the mature person owes its efficiency to the slow and inefficient learning that has gone before. Indeed various physical and mental responses which have at maturity all the properties of a reflex are, in fact, learned over a period of years, the apparent instinctiveness of numerous perceptions is in reality the end result of a long learning process.

Dr. Streff explains that the infinitely complicated and subtle process seems to work like this: every time the visual system receives a stimulus, it analyzes and matches that against the memory bank of cumulative experience of the whole body/mind system. Accordingly, the way it interprets ("sees") that stimulus or image is conditioned by the previous experience of the whole organism. At the same time, the new stimulus is added to and synthesized with the old experience, and becomes a part of the analyzing-matching mechanism that is applied to the next stimulus. Vision is thus a conditioned response. By way of explanation, Professor Samuel Renshaw of Ohio State University has said cryptically that "the stimulus lies within the response," but the paraphrase of Dr. Lawrence Macdonald, a training optometrist of Newton, Massachusetts, is clearer: "We see what we're set to see, what we expect to see. In a sense, the show is over before the curtain goes up."

If vision thus affects development and response (meaning behavior), it follows that a wide range of human failings, defects, and inadequacies—including poor coordination, postural slump, nervous tension, learning difficulties in school or on the job, and the general inability to cope with practical problems of everyday life—are directly related to the visual system. The full development of the brain as a mature and efficient perceiving, thinking, problem-solving mechanism depends on the quality of the information it receives, and this comes mainly from the eyes. Therefore, if the eyes are deficient, poorly coordinated with each other or in relation to other body systems, or adversely affected by stress or bad posture, the brain will almost certainly be performing inefficiently and well below its potential. On the other hand, because the quality of vision is not predetermined and fixed, but is a variable influenced by and influencing the conditions in which it operates, it follows that if the conditions can be changed then the quality of vision can be changed. If the quality of information received through the visual system can be improved, then the efficiency of the brain and indeed of the whole body/mind system can be correspondingly improved.

The following case histories demonstrate that visual training can bring about these results. Sometimes this is accomplished mainly through a better alignment or coordination of the visual and body systems *without* significant improvement in the refractive measurement of the eyes; sometimes there is also substantial optometric improvement. Because the factors in the equation are so numerous and complex, there is, as Dr. Francke has noted, "no one-to-one relationship between refractive measurement and a patient's performance." But with or without optometric improvement, the case histories all show an enhancement of overall performance.

Eliza

Eliza is now 16. As a newborn baby, she needed a small dose of oxygen in the first days of her life, and it was later feared this had caused slight brain damage. In the first grade she was slow to read and to learn the alphabet; this led to a suspicion of dyslexia, which in turn led to her being given some initial eye training: she drew circles on the blackboard with both hands and identified objects in a black bag by touch alone. The training lasted only a few months. Thereafter she developed as an apparently normal child, yet one who was notably sloppy in her reading, writing, and thinking habits. Although she enjoyed reading aloud, she frequently missed or mispronounced words; in mathematics she was plagued by needless errors. Her whole approach to life was slapdash and vague, and she was poorly coordinated physically.

A visual-training optometrist examined her in the spring of 1976 and found that her eyes, although they tested 20/20, were badly discoordinated. He prescribed a range of simple eye exercises with an emphasis on balancing procedures, plus training glasses (rotating prisms) for walking. Eliza took to the training with unexpected enthusiasm and diligence, arising each day before breakfast to do her various exercises and genuinely enjoying her daily three-mile walks in the woods near her home. The training was entirely at home under her mother's supervision, supplemented by visits to the optometrist every six weeks.

A year later, the results were remarkable. She was a notably calmer, more gracious, more contented person. She now spoke fluently and precisely, and her handwriting was much clearer. In school, according to her mother, "she went from booby to star." In mathematics, which she had had great difficulty understanding, she was moved into the fast section of her class. Eliza's art teacher noted with amazement that her drawings had moved from flat, unimaginative two-dimensional renderings to "sophisticated, odd-angled three-dimensional works." In English, she showed a longer attention span and a sharper focus that were reflected in better grammar, better spelling, and a surer grasp of the material under study. In family games, including chess and cards, her parents noticed that she was quicker, more interested, and more alert.

The net result of these changes for Eliza was a greater sense of confidence and a stronger sense of self. As her mother put it, "no more nervous giggling, and a calm rejection of booze and pot in which a number of her contemporaries were beginning to indulge." Always a very pretty child, but rather unnoticed in school because of her vagueness and slowness, she now adjusted to a new popularity.

Eliza's mental efficiency showed dramatic improvement, but the optometric measurements of her eyes changed only slightly.

Tom

Tom was graduated from college in 1967, but never read comfortably or well, was tired most of the time, and earned only average grades. He went to eye doctors who told him there was nothing significantly wrong with his eyes, although he was slightly farsighted and slightly astigmatic. After college he became a computer programmer, but this type of work seemed to aggravate his eye problems, for he suffered general fatigue, a chronic stiff neck, and painful eyestrain after reading for only a few minutes. After four years, he found it so uncomfortable to work under fluorescent light that he wore prescription dark glasses all day long. At that point he went to see a visual-training optometrist.

The doctor found Tom's vision was not severely deficient, but he suffered from an inability to see beyond a given target at both near point and distance. The doctor prescribed training lenses for both reading and distance, classroom training, and home exercises. Tom ran one mile a day five days a week and did supplementary calisthenics, which almost immediately improved his energy level. After two months, he was able to discard his distance glasses. After four months, he experienced a fairly uncomfortable "transition," characterized by headaches and fatigue. But as the transition ended, he was aware that his eyes were considerably improved—he could see more space, control more detail, and carry on his job without significant eyestrain or subsequent fatigue.

The doctor changed Tom's reading glasses to reflect his

new visual range, and three months later he experienced "a transition in my thinking process." His job as manager of customer services in a computer software service bureau required him to shift swiftly from one problem to another, and to suggest technical or procedural solutions over the telephone after listening to a description of the customer's problem. His problem-solving work now became notably swifter and more efficient. Tasks that had taken forty-five minutes he found could now be accomplished in half the time. For about six months, he experienced a fluctuation in efficiency, sometimes reverting to his earlier, lower level of performance, but he eventually stabilized at the new, higher level. Thereafter, he noted a steady and progressive improvement in his intellectual efficiency. "I began thinking in real time, was able to deal immediately with ideas put to me, manipulate and analyze them, and provide immediate responses."

There was also a gain in calmness and self-assurance. Before training, Tom was a tense, clipped, rather uptight personality; now he is resilient in his relations with people. Optometrically, his eyes were not severely deficient when he began the training, but they were poorly aligned with his body systems, with the result that he was stressed and performing well below his apparent potential. The visual training was first directed to reducing stress and tension in his eyes and body, with the aim of recapturing lost energy for more constructive uses. When that goal was achieved, it turned toward a realization of the higher mental efficiency that was being blocked by poor synchronization between the visual and body systems. Tom's subjective feeling of both physical and mental improvement was supported by the optometric measurements.

Jay

Jay is the 12-year-old son of a waitress and an unemployed parking attendant on welfare. In 1974 he was placed in a special class for slow learners. After three years there, his attention span still remained near zero; he could not read, indeed he could not even master the alphabet. His mother was, however, an alert, conscientious woman deeply devoted to helping her son; she felt intuitively that the basic problem was in his eyes. When it became clear to her that he was not making any progress in school, she took him to be tested by a training optometrist.

The doctor found that Jay's eyes were badly coordinated, each one aimed at a different point in space, and that only through great muscular exertion could the boy bring them into focus on the same target. The exertion produced such stress that he could not sustain a binocular focus, and this condition of unstable fusion was the cause of his totally inadequate attention span. In a test designed to simulate depth perception, Jay showed "low stereopsis," which indicates low eye efficiency and, in most cases, low physical and mental coordination as well.

The first training exercise given to Jay was to stand in front of a wall chart on which large block letters were written—80 letters in rows of 10. To simplify the exercise at first, the doctor exposed only one fourth of the chart. Standing before it, Jay was instructed to bounce a playground ball and simultaneously to read aloud one letter at a time, catching the ball after he announced each letter. As his mental-physical coordination gradually improved, he was able to call out the next letter without actually catching the ball, so that bouncing and calling out became a single continuous process. A second exercise for Jay was to stand before a blackboard and draw chalk circles with both hands to the beat of a metronome. Sometimes the instruction was to draw the two circles in the same direction, sometimes in opposite directions; the pace of the metronome was gradually speeded up. A third exercise was to walk back and forth on a four-inch balancing rail, also to the beat of a metronome, while calling out letters on the chart. Sometimes Jay performed this walking exercise with both eyes open; sometimes one of his eyes was covered with an eye patch.

Jay performed these exercises in the doctor's office and then repeated them at home under his mother's guidance together with certain other simple procedures designed to improve the ability of his eyes to shift easily from near to far focus (and vice versa). Because his mother was disciplined and conscientious, and Jay was an agreeable patient, the whole process, while time-consuming, was "no great hassle."

After three months, tests showed a marked improvement in the acuity, depth perception, and coordination of both eyes. Simultaneously Jay began to read at the first-grade level and with this breakthrough he began to manifest a marked change of attitude toward school, learning, and life in general. Whereas he had previously been listless, now he became eager to learn and his interests broadened out to embrace a much wider spectrum of ideas, sports, movies, and friends. His schoolteacher was so impressed with the dramatic change in Jay's performance and attitude that he arranged to pay a visit to the training optometrist during classroom training.

Jay was soon placed part-time in a regular school class. While special schooling will still be required for several more years, there is now real hope that Jay will be able to catch up with his peers. Both parents recognize that, without the improved alignment of his visual and body/mind systems brought about by a program of visual and perceptual training, they would still be without hope for Jay's normal intellectual development. Because of what happened, the family feels a lot of pride. Jay has become a more intelligent, more interested, more energetic, more purposeful boy who is determined to make it on his own.

Philip

A man in his early forties, Philip had the distance vision, depth perception, and hand-eye coordination of a former fighter pilot in the Korean War, and was so good with his hands that he went almost instinctively into the construction business. But, although he enjoyed perfect distance vision and a great deal of energy, he had never (so long as he could remember) been able to read for more than half an hour without losing concentration or actually falling asleep. In the construction business he naturally focused his efforts on supervising building projects in the field, leaving the paper work, which he dreaded, to his partners. His business, his ambition, a growing family to bring up and educate, and a wide range of social and community commitments added up to a strenuous, complicated, and fast-paced life. He appeared to handle the stress well, although he drank a martini with lunch and a bourbon or two before dinner, spoke in a clipped staccato, and gave the impression of being constantly in motion.

In 1977, Philip took one of his children to a visual-training optometrist, and stayed to have his own eyes examined. He had worn reading glasses, but they had not been checked or changed for several years; he had never worn distance glasses. After testing Philip's eyes, the doctor told him he should begin wearing glasses not only for reading but for all other purposes, including driving and athletics. The reason, the doctor explained, was that Philip's eyes were badly coordinated at both the near and middle distances, and that he was exerting tremendous energy to achieve reasonable binocular efficiency in the whole range of his daily activities. Somewhat shocked and surprised by the diagnosis, Philip nevertheless began following the doctor's instructions to the letter. In addition to putting on his general-purpose glasses the moment he stepped out of bed in the morning, and switching to his reading glasses for close work, he took long, fast-paced walks with his daughter, and performed four or five basic training exercises every day. Initially he had trouble with balancing exercises, and his tennis game (which he now played with his general-purpose glasses) turned erratic; there were times when he totally lost sight of the ball above his head and at certain other angles. Also during the first few weeks, his eyes watered a good deal and occasionally felt as though they were filled with sand. The muscles beside and behind them began to feel as though someone were screwing them tighter and tighter, as the lenses pulled them toward a convergence at a shorter distance than before. After two months, he had a "transition" over one weekend. His eyes watered and his head ached. But when things cleared up after twelve hours, he was aware that the world was much brighter and that he was seeing a good deal more of it clearly. The volume of his space intake was much larger. His family suddenly noticed that his eyes, which had been a rather dull slate color, were now bright blue.

He also began to read with greater ease, and over the following weeks found that he could read for four hours at a stretch without any noticeable strain or fatigue. During this same period, he and his partners bought a second construction company. Philip was a prime mover in the negotiations, conducted them with great skill, and in the process spent long hours analyzing written reports and contracts. Both in conducting the merger negotiations and in carrying the new management workload, he was aware of "a great improvement in the quickness of my perception. I can keep a hundred details in my head and bring them out whenever I need them. I can also see the whole picture more clearly, and distinguish more acutely between the important and less important elements of a decision. My sense of timing is better."

In addition to a marked increase in mental efficiency, Philip experienced other improvements from a year of visual training: his whole body/mind system was more relaxed and under better control; no longer feeling the need for it, he gave up hard liquor in all forms, and lost twenty pounds.

VISION AND CULTURE

Culture also shapes vision, for what and how a person sees is also contingent upon the kind of space world he is offered and what perspectives within it are regarded as culturally important. People raised in the city tend to see primarily vertical and horizontal surfaces as compared to the oblique. They also tend to be nearsighted as compared to cowboys and deep-sea fishermen, who are usually farsighted. A Chinese child raised in the crowded city of Shanghai will tend to develop a style of vision that emphasizes near objects; another child, living in the vast Australian outback, will tend to give primary attention to far objects—and he may become a more expansive personality. As a person develops his visual style from the information available to him, he comes to emphasize particular aspects of objects and events and to ignore others. Some individuals organize their universe in great detail, others only in broad outline. What and how a person sees largely determines how he behaves; that is, the kind of real events he routinely pays attention to and the kind of events he routinely ignores define his characteristic behavior.

It is a fact that our modern American, white collar, post-industrial society produces a very large number of nearsighted (myopic) citizens; most specialists in visual care attribute this directly to our strong orientation to such concentrated near-point work as reading, writing, clerical record-keeping, and executive paper-pushing. When confronted daily with close-in visual tasks, often requiring pinpoint acuity to master complicated detail, the eyes show a strong tendency to adjust their point of convergence to the normal distance for reading; this adjustment gradually becomes a set pattern to which the posture and related body rhythms make corresponding compensatory shifts. The net effect is a constriction of the whole body/mind system beginning with the eye muscles. When American children first enter school, only a small percentage of them evidence any significant visual problems —in the first grade, only about one child in ten has a serious visual problem. By the time they reach the sixth grade, however, 25 percent of the boys and 30 percent of the girls are myopic, the difference in incidence between the sexes being attributable to a slightly earlier intellectual development in girls. According to Dr. John Streff, "girls grasp concepts earlier in their development than do boys, but boys catch up in a short time and then generally move ahead. As they do so, their myopia rate goes up."

There continues to be a classic debate as to whether visual problems are hereditary or caused by environment. It is accepted that children whose parents or grandparents have a history of cross-eyedness are somewhat more likely to develop cross-eye and that parents who are myopic are more likely to raise myopic children. But this evidence does not necessarily support the advocates of the hereditary theory. If the child lives in the same surroundings as the parents, and particularly if he participates in the same kind of work and play activities, a style of vision manifesting the same strengths and inefficiencies as the parents' may in fact reflect mainly environmental influences.

Environment and work intensity are major contributing factors. Studies have shown, for example, that intense, high achievers in school are more prone to myopia than their less industrious peers; graduate students have a higher incidence than undergraduates. Submarine crews—especially officers and men in nuclear submarines who stay under water for long periods—are prone to myopia. Monkeys kept in small walled cages develop myopia. And in a recent study of Eskimo families in Alaska, two researchers, Francis A. Young and William Baldwin, found startling visual differences between generations. The parents and grandparents, unschooled hunters and trappers on the vast open tundras, were almost all farsighted and showed virtually no myopia. But of the current generation of Eskimo children, required by Alaskan statehood to attend school regularly, 58 percent were found to be myopic.

Dr. Amiel Francke, in conjunction with anthropologist William K. Carr, conducted an experiment in 1973 to test their assumption that a society's culture—as reflected in its child-rearing practices, educational methods, architecture, furniture, and attitudes toward social organization—definitely affects the way in which the members of that society see and how they interpret what they see. Francke and Carr selected subjects from widely dissimilar cultures—Chinese and American, a choice facilitated by the fact that Carr was a China specialist. The first step was to define aspects of American and Chinese lifestyles that seemed relevant to visual development, and then to compare the differences against the test data.

They noted, for example, that Chinese use chopsticks while Americans use knife and fork. Chinese food is already cut into small pieces, while American food usually requires cutting. These differences lead to different eating positions and a different kind of hand-eye coordination. Also, Chinese writing involves not only the shaping of intricate characters, but also an erect posture because the characters are formed with the writing implement held vertically; conversely, American writing is from left to right and requires the head and torso to be at an angle to the writing surface. Chinese eat and work at higher tables than Americans do, with the result that food, books, work materials, and children's playthings are closer to the eyes. A typical Chinese house is surrounded by a high wall, and the wall is built close to the house; the typical Chinese family thus has limited opportunities for distant viewing.

After analyzing these characteristics (prepared by Carr and a panel of sociologists), Dr. Francke and a panel of two other optometrists predicted that the standard 21-point optometric exam would show that representative Chinese were more visually aware of their immediate surroundings than representative Americans—meaning that they would build their space world inward (toward themselves) from the object they were looking at; at the same time they would be relatively indifferent to distant objects.

The test results bore out the predictions with remarkable accuracy. For example, when eight Chinese were tested for distance acuity, all but one were below normal, within the 20/25 to 20/40 range. As Francke and Carr reported, "when this amount of this acuity loss occurs in Americans, they are usually aware of it and usually seek optometric assistance." But the Chinese, even those who wore no glasses at all, felt their distance vision was perfectly adequate. Distant targets appeared unimportant to them. Americans and Chinese apparently have different attitudes about how sharply one needs to see at a distance. Similarly, in a test where the subject's attention was directed to a chart at a distance of 18 feet, the average convergence point for both Chinese and Americans was short of the chart. But a much higher percentage of the Chinese focused closer than did Americans, and the average point of focus was much closer for the Chinese. In brief, seven of the eight Chinese tested nearsighted as against five of the eight Americans. On the other hand, the Chinese showed an ability to "control" about twice the volume of space inward from a distant target as the Americans showed. The postures of all eight Chinese displayed the expected forward-thrust pelvis and inward-thrust shoulders—the classic posture of the myope.

VISION AS PROCESS

Functional optometry took a great step forward with the introduction and use of cybernetics as a means of explaining how vision functions in relation to various other bodily systems. *Cybernetics,* the term coined by Norbert Weiner in his famous book of the same name, means roughly "steersman." The book developed the theory of feedback as a means of explaining how the functioning of our various complicated subsystems is corrected, refined, and stabilized to assure an efficient performance of the whole body/mind system.

The application of cybernetics to vision constituted a dramatic breakthrough for the functional optometrists of the new school. Observing the feedback process, they were reinforced in their conviction that the visual system is dominant, that it takes the lead in directing and influencing the life of every human. This led them to the conclusion that the body/mind system is a self-directing, self-correcting organism led and mediated largely by the visual system through a continuous process of adjustment. They recognized that other senses, especially the auditory and the tactile, play important roles in providing and processing useful information, but watching the feedback process at work, they were convinced that all other senses are inferior to vision in terms of the qualitative capacity to receive and process information.

It was about this time, between 1948 and 1950, that Dr. Gesell was preparing to make his pronouncement that vision is always a process, and indeed a learning process. And it was then that Skeffington declared, somewhat more definitively, that the *main purpose of vision is to process information*—that is, to select and develop from the billions of stimuli presented to the retina and the brain those items of information that will help the organism to survive, build its knowledge of the world, correct its mistakes, and reach the goals it has set for itself. These developments led in turn to a new emphasis in visual training on achieving goals based on the needs and desires expressed by the patient. For example, Dr. Robert Kraskin of Washington, D.C., developed a visual-training program in the 1950s organized around goals ranging widely from major life challenges (like successful completion of law school or entrance into a military academy) to enhanced social pleasures (like playing a better game of golf). Dr. Kraskin urged the patient to keep his personal goal in mind at all times while performing any visual exercise or activity, and to discover for himself how that might be used to improve his total performance in relation to the stated goal.

SPACE/TIME RELATIONSHIPS

Cybernetics and the concept of vision as a continuous feedback process also focused new attention on the importance of accurately handling space/time relationships.

What is a space/time relationship? As applied to visual training, it means the form, shape, size, and movement of objects perceived by the visual system (if an object seen is stationary, then the time component is the time required for the viewer to move to the object). The term "space/time" suggests that space and time are different but interchangeable ways of measuring the *same phenomenon*. Time is often expressed in terms of space or distance, and distance is often expressed in terms of time. Question: "How long will it take me to walk to the grocery store?" Answer: "It's about a quarter of a mile." Conversely: "How far is the store?" Answer: "About ten minutes by automobile." Space and time are interchangeable because the fundamental fact of our existence is that all life involves movement through space at varying rates of speed—that is, elapsed time. The world we live in is not stationary, nor can we control the movement of most other objects in it. We must learn therefore to make accurate judgments about the nature and the relationships of objects moving at various speeds through space, so that (at a simple level) we can survive and (at a higher level) we can become more efficient, accomplish more, and find greater satisfaction in life. This rule applies to both physical coordination and the act of thinking.

For example, we walk down streets and through rooms in which other people are standing or moving, and we find that life is more efficient if we can avoid bumping into them. People who possess reasonably good brain-eye-hand-foot coordination gravitate naturally to games involving moving objects—balls, pucks, shuttlecocks, and other human players —and they move efficiently through countless space/time tasks without being fully aware of their complexity. But people without that kind of good coordination are usually poor at making judgments in space/time, and they usually adapt their lifestyles to their performance. They will not, for example, play games with moving balls, but will become hikers, campers, or swimmers, or will seek out nonathletic recreation that does not require precise spatial judgments. They may refrain from driving cars or shopping in busy supermarkets. The essential difference between those who handle physical space/time relationships well and those who handle them poorly lies both in the quality of their visual perceptions and the way in which they are able to translate these into efficient body/mind responses.

Dr. Albert Shankman, a training optometrist of Norwalk, Connecticut, also distinguishes between what he terms internal and external time. The first is your personal sense or judgment of time—for example, how long is a minute? how long is an hour? The second is real time as measured by the clock. Dr. Shankman has found from his training practice that, where disparity between the patient's internal time and external time is great, his performance in the real world is apt to be uncoordinated, inefficient, out of synch. In short, the patient hasn't got it together.

Given the pervasive interaction between the eyes and the brain, it is not surprising that there should be a direct correlation between a person's ability to handle space/time relationships in the physical world and his ability to think. Better control of physical space/time leads directly to better mental coordination—that is, to a more efficient organization of the whole intellectual process, from perception to creativity to problem solving—*because the fundamental unit of thinking is space/time.* Space and time being almost completely interchangeable in cerebral action, space/time relationships are the building blocks of thought. *Stated differently, abstract intellectual thought is based upon the elementary physical space/time relationships perceived mainly by the eyes, and upon the progressive organization, interpretation, and manipulation of these perceptions by the brain.*

As a viewing person, you form a space/time relationship with an object in your field of vision whenever you ask and answer the questions "Where is it?" "What is it?" From childhood onward you progressively build your own "space world," as we have earlier explained, by what Dr. Gesell called "an exquisite and minute process," furnishing what was originally empty space (in a perceptual, behavioral sense) with the data bank of all your cumulative experience. Gradually you see similarities and develop relationships between images and objects; later you use words to represent the things themselves; finally you learn to "manipulate" the word symbols in various combinations, which is the process of thinking. Dr. John Streff points out that the ability to think creatively requires more than getting a single clear perception of a cluster of ideas. Rather, it requires a sufficient flexibility of the visual system to "see" the components of the cluster in different ways, in different combinations, and from various angles or points of view. Dr. Shankman agrees: "The skill of seeing relationships is a principal object of visual training." He adds that "visual training is essentially brain training."

From their clinical experience with patients, leading visual-training optometrists have concluded that, where this flexibility is not present in the visual system, the person will show a tendency to think in set patterns and to lack imagination. Open-mindedness, creativity, and deeper understanding depend on the ability to move ideas around, visually and mentally, in order to arrive at new combinations that were not initially apparent.

Visual perceptions of space/time are thus the building blocks of thought. It follows logically that, as you improve your ability to identify, locate, and interpret the physical components in your field of vision, you also improve your ability to manipulate the symbolic, intellectual superstructure.

Dr. Francke uses a test that rather precisely illustrates this visual-cerebral interaction and the organizing power of vision. Here doctor and patient sit opposite each other at a small table; each has before him a matching set of children's blocks varying in shape and color. While the patient closes his eyes, the doctor arranges his own blocks in a particular pattern. He then shuts off the patient's view with a large

63

sheet of cardboard. When all is in readiness, the doctor instructs the patient to focus his eyes on the spot where the pattern will appear when the cardboard is lifted. He then lifts and lowers the cardboard very quickly, allowing the patient about one fifth of a second to view the pattern. The patient then attempts to duplicate the pattern he has seen by gathering his own blocks and putting them down on the table one at a time. He is not allowed to rearrange any block after it has touched the surface of the table. The patient's mental efficiency in this case is a direct consequence of his visual efficiency. The quality of his eyesight—that is, the quality of his attitude of perceptual readiness directed to physical objects in space—determines what and how much he sees and how well he is able to re-create the pattern of images in his mind and subsequently on the table.

VISION AND THE COMPUTER

Computers are of great value because of their huge memory-storage capacity and phenomenally fast response. A large modern computer has a memory capacity of about one million words, and its "switching time" is measured in nano-seconds (a nanosecond is equivalent to one billionth of a second, the time it takes light to travel about a foot). It takes a computer 30 nanoseconds to complete a loop—that is, to comprehend and respond to a specific problem.

Dr. Lawrence W. Macdonald has carried the concepts of feedback and information processing in human vision a step farther by developing a comparison between the operation of a computer and the operation of the eye-brain system. That they can legitimately be compared is shown by the fact that, despite the size of modern computers' storage capacity, the memory capacity of the human brain is estimated to be two and a half times greater.

With regard to the speed of response, the computer is, of course, way ahead. Compared to the computer's 30 nanoseconds, human response time varies between 150 and 300 milliseconds. Dr. Skeffington concluded that the average human response time is 200 milliseconds, or about one fifth of a second. He also concluded that, if we cannot grasp the task at hand in one fifth of a second, we have to run the information through a second time. And if comprehension is still lacking, we must break the task down into smaller units that are comprehensible within the one-fifth second response time. After comprehension of the smaller unit is achieved, we must then reassemble the units in an attempt to grasp the larger concept.

Although the computer response time is much faster than our own, Dr. Macdonald argues that the human visual system can ingest a larger number of information items. Information comes to the computer in the form of a coded punch card or magnetic tape. Information comes to humans through the senses—primarily through the visual system. A large modern computer can process thirty-two information items in one input cycle (30 nanoseconds), but the human visual system can process 100 million information items in one input cycle (one fifth of a second). This is the capacity of *each* retina, but Dr. Macdonald believes we must assume that our "binocular visual system is redundant"—that is, that the two retinas in effect process the same items of information. This is in fact necessary if the eyes are coordinating with each other and thus making sense of what is processed.

Within the framework of this general computer analogy,

Dr. Macdonald has introduced the concept of "microprocessing," which he relates to the flexibility of response, or fine tuning, in the visual system that is a major goal of visual training. It is precisely such flexibility and versatility in the motor-sensory functioning of the visual system that produces good balance, smooth coordination, and good rhythm and timing in both mental and physical activities. In computer technology, a microcompressor is an integrated circuit designed to perform one step in a series of logical functions. It is part of a larger whole and is directed by the master control mechanism to perform a particular task (a microprocess). Dr. Macdonald argues that the goal of visual training is to increase the number and efficiency of "microcompressors"— meaning an increased capacity for refinement and sublety in visual response—within the whole body/mind system because the greater the number and variety of these, the greater will be the range and flexibility of response to any given situation. Many years ago, Dr. Skeffington noted varying "degrees of freedom" in the visual systems of his patients. Where there was relative rigidity or constriction of perception (as in near-sightedness), the patient was capable of only an average, inflexible physical response or a correspondingly unimaginative mental response to a given stimulus or challenge. On the other hand, the patient who showed a flexible ability to "accommodate" both near and far objects, and whose peripheral vision was strong, was capable of a much wider range of physical response and was usually able to come to a decision more quickly and efficiently. Dr. Macdonald thus argues that the development of a larger number of "microcompressors" is a principal goal of visual training because they contribute directly to a more efficient performance in every aspect of life.

The computer flow-chart analogy to visual information processing is valuable for several reasons: it points up the essential continuity of the function, and makes it possible to define visual defects and difficulties as a resistance to the flow, like a log placed in the middle of a stream that slows the flow of water. Visual training thus becomes a technique for "troubleshooting" to locate and identify these resistance points, and then to take remedial measures that will restore the processing to the ideal condition of unobstructed information flow.

The swift operational flow of the visual system is, of course, frequently slowed or blocked by a number of different "logs" in various parts of the muscular or nervous systems, throughout the body. The visual system will adjust to these adverse conditions by trying to neutralize or bypass them, and the result will be a performance of relative inefficiency. If the conditions are serious, the adjustments may well involve adverse compensatory postural shifts and thus corresponding changes in eyesight. Basically, according to Dr. Macdonald, we have the choice of making structural or functional adjustments to the defects, or ceasing to function—that is, giving up, going to bed, or dying. Because visual training is addressed to the problem of correcting and improving the "lead system," the master coordinator for the organism as a whole, it is perhaps uniquely positioned to bring about a correction of the adverse conditions—be they backaches or nervous tension—by restoring a harmonious alignment of the whole body/mind system.

Five

The Importance of Reducing Stress

INDIVIDUAL HUMAN DEVELOPMENT is always a chancy process because it depends on such variables as genetic endowment, nutrition, cultural background, quality of schooling, and personal motivation. The same is true with regard to the quality of visual development and performance. As we have seen, an individual's visual "space world" is a plastic, flexible domain that undergoes continuous change and expansion as his visual system grows from infancy to childhood and from youth to maturity. But the child's visual system may develop in irregular patterns, rhythms, and unforeseen directions, and it will be decisively influenced by bodily health, the pace of life, and the physical and emotional stresses imposed by the particular environment.

An extremely important purpose, indeed a central feature, of the new visual training is the reduction or elimination of stress—which is defined as the general wear and tear on the body caused by the body's response to abnormal conditions or demands. The new school holds that defective vision is by definition stressful vision, because the body/mind system must expend extra energy to overcome the defects and achieve a sufficient degree of binocular efficiency to accomplish life's basic tasks. Moreover, as we noted in the discussion of posture and vision, the body's effort to compensate for defective eyesight leads to postural tension and thence to postural deviations that produce a variety of ailments, including neck pain, backaches, pinched nerves, and menstrual irregularities.

Dr. Hans Selye, perhaps the one great authority on the subject, has defined stress as the nonspecific response of the body and mind to any challenge or threat to the organism; also as the "struggle for the self-preservation (or homeostasis) of parts within the whole." His findings have demonstrated that stress is measurable—by adrenal enlargement, increased cortical concentration in the blood, loss of weight, and other indicators—and he has labeled the sum of such changes the "general adaptation syndrome," or G.A.S. It develops in three stages: (1) the alarm reaction, which is the immediate bodily response to a wound, infection, or mental shock; (2) the stage of resistance, in which the body fights back through the nervous and endocrine (hormonal) systems to maintain its structural integrity and steady-state functioning; and (3) the stage of exhaustion, in which the body has no more energy left to fight against the causes of the stress—at which point it either surrenders or is given a reprieve by removal of the causes.

For purposes of the new school approach to visual training, the following is fundamental: Dr. Selye concluded that every living being is endowed with only so much adaptive energy or vitality. It varies widely in individuals, being in part a matter of genetic heritage, but it is finite in each case.

Accordingly, stress caused by postural distortion or defective vision will siphon off large or small amounts of this finite adaptive energy by requiring the body/mind system to work harder merely to get through each ordinary day. Such waste means that the person either operates at a lower level of energy or ages faster, and may lack the reserve strength to meet sustained physical or mental crises.

"Physiologic aging," Dr. Selye has said, "is not determined by the time elapsed since birth, but by the total amount of wear and tear to which the body has been exposed." There is accordingly a great difference between physiologic and chronologic age. "One man may be much more senile in body and mind, and much closer to the grave, at 40 than another at 60; true age depends largely on the rate of wear and tear, on the speed of self-consumption; for life is essentially a process which gradually spends the given amount of adaptive energy we inherited from our parents." Dr. Selye likens vitality to a special kind of bank account that you can use up by withdrawals but cannot increase by deposits. Your only control over this precious fortune is the rate at which you make your withdrawals. The solution is not to stop withdrawing, for that would be death; nor is it to withdraw just enough for survival, for that would permit only a vegetative life worse than death. "The intelligent thing to do," Selye has written, "is to withdraw and expend generously but never wastefully for worthless efforts." Stress is not all bad. It is both positive and negative. It is experienced when we suffer intense physical injury or mental anguish, but also when we alert our senses to cross a busy intersection or play a hard tennis match, or when we feel sheer exhilaration. But it is the efficient or inefficient expenditure of this finite resource that makes all the difference.

While all adaptive energy is finite, Dr. Selye believes it

may break down into two distinct categories, which can lead to good and bad consequences. When "superficial" adaptive energy is exhausted through exertion, it can be slowly restored from "deeper reserves" by rest. This is "good" in the sense that it lends a certain resilience to our response to stress; it also protects us from wasting adaptive energy too lavishly, for acute fatigue automatically stops us. It is "bad" in the sense that our ability to restore this "superficial" adaptive energy from the "deeper reserves" may trick us into the careless optimism of believing we have made good our loss. Actually, there has been a net depletion. Among the many autopsies he has performed, Dr. Selye claims never to have seen a person who died of old age in the sense that all the organs of the body had worn out proportionately, merely by having been used too long. This is not what happens. "We invariably die because one vital part has worn out too early in proportion to the rest of the body. Life, the biologic chain that holds our parts together, is only as strong as its weakest vital link." Yet even recognizing the finite nature of adaptive energy, Dr. Selye believes we can significantly lengthen the average human life span by living in better harmony with natural laws.

Whether we should lead a slow or rapid, colorful or bland existence is not entirely within our choosing, for the optimum tempo at which we are to consume life is largely inherited from our predecessors. Yet even though inborn aptitudes form the base line of our adaptability, "the manifest features" of a person's character and physical appearance are largely the result of the way in which this innate adaptability has responded to the stresses imposed during the individual's own lifetime. Within broad limits, each person, through the exercise of willpower, discipline, and wisdom of choice, can act to determine the thrust, character, and span of his life.

Each person, Dr. Selye has said, is like a pilot who has left the ground in an airplane. Unless he wants to kill himself, he cannot stop the motor for a nice long rest before he gets back to earth. He has a given airplane and a given fuel supply, and there is the inexorable fact of gravity. But he can fly at a speed and on a course best suited to his machine under the prevailing weather conditions. Similarly with each human being. He cannot stop after being born, unless he wants to die, yet he can do much through voluntary choice of conduct to get as far as possible with a given bodily structure and a given supply of adaptive energy. For example, he can live and express his personality at a tempo and in directions best suited to his inherited talents under the prevailing social conditions. "The great art," Selye wrote, "is to express our vitality through the particular channels and at the particular speed which nature foresaw for us. . . . The human body—like the tires of a car or the rug on a floor—wears longest when it wears evenly." Thousands of people, consciously or unconsciously, use caffeine, tobacco, alcohol, and other drugs to extend their energies artificially. The inexorable fact is that this process accelerates the drawing down of finite energy reserves and thus virtually assures that they will burn out faster than necessary.

STRESS AND VISION

There is obviously a connection here between the stress factor and the new school of visual training: the person with defective vision or postural distortion must expend extra adaptive energy every day, leaving fewer reserves (or none at all) for sustained physical or mental crises, creative achievement, or the enjoyment of a robust recreation. Life is difficult and may be short. Yet if the visual defects and postural warps can be removed or balanced out through an effective visual-training program, then stress can be reduced, and life can be healthier, longer, and lived at a higher level of efficiency and satisfaction.

A number of studies have convincingly demonstrated that intensive "near-point vision work," such as reading, writing, and related desk activity—the kind of work that pervades and dominates our post-industrial white-collar society— generates stress, which in turn produces a constriction of the visual system. This is both a physical and mental phenome-non. The eyes do not change structure, and the retina con-tinues to receive as many undifferentiated stimuli as ever. But, as Dr. Streff has noted, when you tighten any muscle (in the eye or the leg), you lose feedback and thus information and awareness. What happens in visual constriction is that less information is processed—that is, synthesized, unified, understood—by the eyes and the brain.

Such findings have been confirmed by measuring the con-stricting effect of stress on visual performance with a retino-scope, an instrument that records various levels of light intensity in the eyes when the organism confronts a variety of situations. For example, when the patient is relaxed and reading for pleasure at his own pace, the retinoscope records whitish pink; when he is required to absorb more difficult material and an understanding of it is within his capability, the retinoscope will record a true pink; when the patient is frustrated by his inability to cope with the material, the retinoscope records a bright red or reddish pink; finally, when the patient loses all rapport with the problem, it shows a dull brick red.

EYE POWER

In one test, Dr. Amiel Francke asks the patient to begin multiplying in his head two times two times two times two— to infinity. Invariably, the retinoscope undergoes a swift progressive change of color, as the patient's mind approaches the "frustration" and then the "wipe-out" levels, indicating his inability to cope any longer with the calculations. It is thus possible, in the space of a minute or so, to observe all of the possible variations in reflex as the patient goes from relaxed calculation into a stress response, which is a constriction of the visual system. If the stress is sustained, it leads in almost every case to semi-permanent visual distortions, chief among which is nearsightedness (myopia). There are three principal reactions to stress. The first is to go into myopia, which closes out the wider world, but adjusts the body/mind system to cope with a large volume of near-point work; the second is to internalize the stress throughout the various body systems, which leads to a variety of physical ailments, including stiff neck and backaches; the third is to drop out entirely—for example, to leave school or quit a job because of a felt inability to cope with the pressures. Dr. Shankman believes that the choice of reaction is an accurate reflection of character. Going into myopia is usually the most intelligent, least destructive response, especially for scholars and others who do close work.

Other studies have shown that this kind of stress response not only constricts the visual system, but also produces similar effects on *all forms of perception,* with far-reaching implications for total comprehension and personality. People restrict their whole sensory performance under stress—they literally see less, hear less, and become less efficient. Fear frequently induces statements such as "I was so scared I didn't hear what he said." Soldiers, anxious and fearful under the stress of battle, often develop a kind of "tunnel vision" that markedly decreases their general perception and efficiency. Indeed, a narrowing of perception, in which the individual under stress unconsciously "turns off" and is no longer aware of many aspects of a given situation, is perhaps the most characteristic response to anxiety. The organism seeks to wall itself off from the threat or trouble with which it cannot fully cope. It follows that physical stress caused by inefficient eyes or bad posture leads, directly or indirectly, both to a constriction of the visual system and to a reduced efficiency of the whole body/mind system.

A program of visual training involving not only eye procedures, but also exercises designed to improve posture, balance, and body awareness is thus a key to the relief of stress and to the achievement of higher levels of energy and of overall performance. A few summaries of actual case histories will serve to underline the truth of this proposition.

Henrietta

Henrietta, aged 23, is a market researcher who suffered severe headaches, double vision, and failing depth perception primarily as a result of intensive typing and clerical work. She wore bifocal glasses, but they gave her no significant relief. As a child of 8, she had undergone a short period of visual training for a condition known as alternating convergence (esotropia) in which the eyes turn in one at a time, but in no consistent pattern. Thereafter she had tried to wear contact lenses, but they caused excessive eyestrain.

She went to see another training optometrist in 1977 who diagnosed a *"tendency* to alternating convergence" (esophoria)—meaning that she could now control her childhood

75

condition by muscular exertion. Ironically this caused her to suffer greater stress than she had known as a child. She had special difficulty in maintaining a steady gaze: the image went from clear to blurred and back again, repeatedly. Owing to these several deficiencies, she had a "fragile binocularity."

She started regular classroom sessions twice a week, supplemented by a variety of home training exercises, all aimed at strengthening and stabilizing her binocularity. The classroom procedures involved the use of lenses and prisms to break down and change the inadequate adaptations and adjustments she had developed in response to her visual disorder. After the first month she felt she was seeing better with less effort, and that her three-dimensional sense was stronger, especially in the morning when her energy was fresh. She was able to judge distances more accurately while driving a car.

Through the use of a training device called "polaroid lenses," which orient each eye in a separate way, she was able to sustain a steady gaze—both eyes processing information simultaneously—for thirty seconds and then for a full minute.

After the second month of training, her sense of the third dimension was greatly strengthened, and she also began to notice small spatial differences, such as crooked pictures on a wall. She could read for longer periods without stress, she could translate distances more accurately into feet and yards, and she discovered a new joy in shopping (in supermarkets and department stores) because each item or piece of merchandise now stood out sharply, individual and discrete. She went to a hockey game and was delighted to discover that she could follow the puck at all times. After the third month, she achieved a much stronger ability to shift focus from near to far and vice versa, and her visual system had stabilized to a point where tension and job stress did not adversely affect her eyesight. "At the end of a hard day, my eyes used to blur after one drink. Now they don't at all."

After five months, her energy level was measurably higher and she needed less sleep. After six months, her visual problem was essentially resolved. The training had substantially corrected the esophoria: her eyes no longer had a tendency to turn in; therefore she did not have to exert muscular energy to prevent the turning. With this correction had come a new sense of strength, energy, and self-confidence. Her whole system was in a more harmonious alignment.

Martin

Martin is 58 years old, short, overweight, and has a poor posture. He is a supervising draftsman in a large architectural firm. When he came to the visual training optometrist in 1977, he could read for only ten minutes at a time; after that, his eyes began to burn and he suffered from tension and fatigue. He wore bifocals with a "base down" prism to correct a tendency of the right eye to gaze upwards (a condition known as hyperphoria). Because his work involved close attention to written detail for long periods of time, Martin was afraid he would lose his job to a younger man.

The doctor found that Martin had several visual deficiencies in addition to the hyperphoria. He could not follow a moving object with both eyes—the eyes jerked instead of following smoothly along the path of movement; he also had poor ability to shift focus from near to far (and vice versa), and he could not sustain a binocular focus at short distances.

77

When he read aloud he often skipped words. He had poor hand-eye coordination, poor peripheral vision, and his handwriting was nearly illegible. This diagnosis indicated that his whole body/mind system suffered from severe chronic stress.

Martin's personal history indicated that he had always learned more through listening than through seeing; he could obtain more information by attending a lecture than by reading the same material in a book. Owing to a brilliant memory, he retained most of what he heard.

In classroom training the doctor concentrated on exercises that used training lenses to develop Martin's ability to focus more steadily, at both near and far, as well as on exercises to strengthen his ability to achieve a binocular fusion. The doctor found that one of Martin's eyes saw things faster than the other, causing information to reach the brain faster from one side, thus producing discoordination and stress. Home training therefore emphasized procedures with one eye patched, in order to train each eye to process information at the same rate of speed. These included the Pencil and Straw exercise "on the Z axis"—meaning an effort to stab the pencil into the straw with the open end of the straw facing the patient (see chapter 7).

After three months Martin became aware of objects at the periphery of his vision, and could do close work for forty-five minutes without fatigue. After the ninth training month he could read comfortably for long periods and had lost all conscious sense of time limits on his reading. He could also play racquetball, which reflected a considerable improvement in hand-eye coordination. The doctor gave him reading glasses, but no distance glasses, and eliminated the "base down" prism. After the tenth month, all of Martin's original symptoms of pain and stress were gone, and he had regained confidence in his ability to hold his job.

Harold

Harold was 10 years old, large for his age and overweight, and without good rapport with his peers, who found him irritating and clumsy. He was hyperactive with a very short attention span and an inability to concentrate. Although he could read, the page frequently blurred, and he lagged far behind his classmates in both speed and comprehension. His eyes tired quickly, whether he was reading or using them for card games, and he refused to participate in sports.

The training optometrist to whom he was brought by his parents found that Harold's basic problem was poor binocular coordination—his eyes did not work well together—aggravated by nearsightedness (myopia). This combination of deficiencies prevented Harold from sustaining a clear binocular focus at either near point or distance. While he could achieve such a focus for brief periods, he could maintain acuity only by stressful straining and squinting; hence, the hypertension, irritability, brief attention span, eye fatigue, and limited comprehension.

He began regular classroom training procedures, supplemented by home exercises. These consisted of walking on a balancing rail while reading letters on a chart in front of him, tipping a balance board back and forth to the beat of a metronome while reading the same letter chart, and lying on the floor while following a moving ball suspended from the ceiling and simultaneously doing certain verbal problems aloud—such as reciting the alphabet forward and backward.

The doctor also gave him bifocal lenses with a low plus for close work to ease him out of his myopia, but with plain clear glass for distance. On his own initiative, Harold started jogging and began to lose weight.

Within four months, Harold realized measurable improvements in every aspect of his life. His binocular coordination greatly improved, and this eliminated both blurred vision and eye fatigue. His attention span grew longer, and he began to read books outside of school on his own initiative. His handwriting became clearer. His comprehension improved, as evidenced by higher marks in English and mathematics. His schoolteacher, who did not know he was taking visual training, remarked to his parents that she "didn't know what had got into Harold because he is doing so much better."

After six months, there was also a marked reduction in his restlessness, so that he became a calmer, more stable personality, and this led in turn to better relations with his peers. His mother noted that Harold was "now a nicer person" and that "other children now call him out to play basketball, which never happened before." He has taken on responsibility for a newspaper route and is conducting every aspect of his life with greater self-confidence.

Bradshaw

Bradshaw is a free-lance writer who suffered severe insomnia over the past ten years and had reached a point of acute depression and frustration when, by chance, he happened to sit next to Ann Hoopes at a Washington dinner party and was thus introduced to the philosophy of the new school functional optometry. Let him tell his own story.

"For years I had been waking up at three or four in the morning, still tired but unable to go back to sleep, feeling tension through my arms and upper body, squirming and twisting in a miserable state until it was necessary to get up at seven. It always took me an hour or more to shake off the fatigue and irritation of the night. I couldn't recall having had what I would call a good night's sleep (meaning six or seven hours straight) more than two or three times a year. Also, I suffered a painful stiffness in my back upon arising, which led to my getting a carpenter in to raise the level of the bathroom sink so I could shave in reasonable comfort. I couldn't bend over far enough. Fortunately, being a strong and energetic person, I could get through the day, but it took conscious pushing much of the time.

"The arthritis clinic at the local hospital checked me out; so did an orthopedic surgeon. They found nothing and recommended back exercises. I did these for a few years, but they did nothing to improve my sleep. My family doctor suggested psychoanalysis, which I rejected; he also prescribed one sleeping pill after another, but these only made me heavy-headed in the morning, and I finally gave them up in disgust. A year or two ago I settled down to pretending my condition was 'normal' or in any event something that had to be accepted as part of my life.

"In July 1977, I had a particularly long stretch of bad sleep, which made me snappier than usual with my children and so adversely affected my tennis game that I promised myself never to play seriously again until I got back into decent physical shape. After anguished consultation with my wife, I even decided to submit myself to a 'sleep clinic,' which I had read about, and was on the point of making definite plans for this when that same evening I happened, by chance, to be seated next to Ann Hoopes. She gave me an earful about the new visual training, and I figured it was worth a try.

"The doctor received me for an hour on August 8. After

81

EYE POWER

an examination, he told me that one of my eyes focused at a twenty-two inches from the target, while the other focused at least five inches closer. The effort expended to make the two eyes work in tandem—achieve what is called binocular fusion—was generating the strain that was giving me insomnia. I had worn rather low-power reading glasses twenty years before, as a response to headaches, but otherwise had never worn glasses. In the various vision tests given me in school and the military, the technician had always put me down as 20/20. The doctor recommended, for openers, that I begin wearing glasses that would bring the farsighted eye to focus at the same distance as the near eye. But rather than make the total correction all at once, he suggested that we try to achieve it in three successive stages: I would wear moderately corrective lenses for one month; then a stronger pair for a second month; then a still stronger pair of glasses for the third month, which would complete the correction. Then he would test my eyes again. I was to wear the glasses only for reading.

"The first day I wore the new glasses, I got a severe headache, felt queasy, and suffered the usual insomnia. But in just a few days, in less than a week, I began to sleep better than I had slept in seven or eight years. Either I would sleep straight through to five or six in the morning (once or twice even to seven), or, if I woke up at three, I was able to go back to sleep easily with little or no twisting and squirming. I even did some dreaming between four and seven o'clock, and dreaming usually means you are coming out of a 'deep sleep'—virtually unprecedented for me. Moreover, I began to be suffused with a feeling of pleasant well-being during the day. I lost the hard edge of resentment and irritability that I had developed in recent years, perhaps at the prospect of having to face yet another sleepless night. My morning back strain virtually faded away. Most exciting of all, I enjoyed some phenomenal bursts of creativity; whereas I usually write one short piece a day—or at most two on very heavy days—there were several times in August, just a few weeks after I started wearing the first pair of glasses, when I wrote with an unprecedented productivity and fluency, and met all the deadlines with time left over.

"The results have not been entirely consistent; I continue to awake at different hours and, although the general level of my sleep is deeper, some nights are better than others. Variables intrude: one night, after some difficult night driving had given me a headache, I slept quite badly; on another night while on vacation, in a strange and uncomfortable bed, I also slept badly. Still, on balance, I am absolutely delighted. It seems reasonable to anticipate further gains—less stress and better sleep, and thus more control of my coordination, energy, and creativity. I find the prospect quite thrilling."

Many manifestations of chronic stress—that is, stress that results from inharmonious coordination or poor alignment of various body systems, rather than that caused by a sudden outside threat—do not at first seem related to vision and the eyes; nor is training and correction of the visual system generally recognized as a central path to a solution to stress problems. However, the experience of the new school training optometrists has shown, time and again, that there is in most cases a direct link between the visual system and stress, no matter in what form the stress may be manifest. This is true, according to Dr. John Streff, because "vision is a neurological balancing system for the whole organism; it engages not only the central nervous system, which controls our voluntary functions, but also the autonomic nervous system, which controls a wide range of involuntary functions." This statement makes the fundamental point we have made before—that vision is the "lead system," the master coordinator, affecting and affected by every other component of the body/mind system.

Six

Essential Elements of Visual Training

A VISUAL TRAINING PROGRAM is similar in some ways to training programs designed to achieve greater proficiency in a range of other specialized fields—for example, music, football, or the military art. Each of these involves discipline and hard work on the part of the trainee, but it also requires supervision—by a master, a coach, a top sergeant —if the training is to produce the desired result. All training of every kind, whether designed to produce pianists, football players, or soldiers, involves the deliberate, judicious application of stress. There is no other known way to stretch the capacity of the trainee, teach him new skills, and raise his level of performance. In a true sense, the trainee must force himself and teach himself, yet he cannot be fully effective without a supervisor. This seeming paradox applies equally to visual training. It cannot be a do-it-yourself program, yet it is, in Dr. Macdonald's words, "a self-monitoring, self-directing, and self-correcting" process involving "a tremendous personal participation on the part of the patient."

The first step must always be a diagnosis of the problem by a professional visual-training optometrist, followed by the design of a training program aimed at correcting the patient's particular visual deficiencies and related problems. The program will usually contain elements of both classroom (i.e., directly supervised) training and home (i.e., guided but unsupervised) training. New school practitioners differ in the emphasis they place upon these closely related aspects of training, but in nearly every case more time is allocated to home training. Dr. Shankman, for example, sees his patients once a week, but expects them to do thirty minutes of training at home each day. Dr. Francke sees his patients twice a week, but assigns them at least an hour a day of home training (more if walking or jogging time is counted). Some patients live at great distances from their optometrists and see them only once every six or eight weeks; their training is thus almost entirely done at home. The same situation applies to most young children; usually they are given home procedures to do under the supervision of their parents, and see their optometrist at infrequent intervals.

A number of fairly standard eye exercises, balancing procedures, and related training techniques—most of them deriving from the workshops, studies, and debates of the Optometric Extension Program—are used by most training optometrists, and we describe some of these later in this chapter. Some practitioners have devised their own variants of these, or have invented and applied a set of new and different techniques. Each training optometrist prescribes his own mix of classroom and home procedures, tailored to the particular problems and capacities of each patient, but there appears to be no sharp distinction between those exercises performed in the classroom and those performed at home, except in one area of overriding importance—lenses. Exercises with lenses are almost always performed in the classroom under close professional supervision. We discuss the special importance of lenses in chapter 8.

The leading practitioners of the new school sometimes differ from one another on particular training techniques, and on the degree of severity involved in their practice, consequences, and side-effects. Most, however, agree on the three fundamental purposes of training. These are:

1. to dislodge the patient from the present visual-postural set that is causing his inefficient performance;
2. to get his body/mind system moving in the desired direction;
3. to achieve a higher quality of visual performance and the improved visual-postural adjustment needed to sustain it.

To meet the first basic purpose, the new school practitioners seek to demonstrate to the patient that there are inconsistencies between what he knows the real world to be like and the way he sees it.

To meet the second and third basic purposes, they employ a variety of procedures designed to achieve better body awareness, better body balance and coordination, the taking in of "more space" through the eyes, improvement in the perception of "size constancy," and greater range, smoothness, and flexibility in the eyes' response to visual tasks.

This chapter endeavors to describe and explain these

essential elements and methods of the new visual training. A range of training exercises, each designed to move the patient toward one of the above specific goals, will be described in chapter 7.

INCONSISTENCIES AND MISMATCHES

A primary purpose of visual training is to "rematch" the visual coordinates with the body coordinates, which means, according to Dr. Lawrence Macdonald, "getting patients to take a hard, fresh look at what they actually see, and to face up to the inconsistencies and mismatches." For example, most people with deficient vision make a conscious effort to believe that the world they see is consistent with the reality they know intellectually—that vertical lines, for example, are truly vertical, not slightly curved; and that the table across the room is really three feet high, not five feet. Frequently, maintaining a sense of consistency requires the suspension of judgment, a suppression of the subconscious awareness that there are in fact disturbing inconsistencies between what you see and what you know to be the reality. To avoid unsettling implications with which they cannot or do not wish to cope, most people resist facing these inconsistencies.

A patient undergoing an eye test may thus report to the optometrist that the wall of the room before him appears to be about three feet high, even though he is aware that when he stands up the ceiling is two feet above his head, so that it must be about eight feet high. When the patient is then asked if the ceiling and the floor appear perfectly horizontal and do not converge toward each other at any point, and he replies in the affirmative, then the optometrist confronts him with the fact of the discrepancy: if the ceiling and floor appear to be horizontal, but the wall looks only three feet high, how then, he asks, does the patient account for the missing five feet of space between the three-foot wall and the floor and ceiling? Thus confronted, the patient must face up explicitly to the truth that the way he sees the world through his eyes is not the world as it really is.

In another example, the optometrist asks the patient to try to focus his eyes on a target ten feet away. The patient seeks to comply and sincerely believes he is doing exactly what is asked, but the testing machine shows that his eyes are actually converging at a distance of twenty-two inches.

Unable to avoid the inconsistency, the patient suffers a temporary disorientation sometimes called "critical empathy" (Ann Hoopes's own experience was described in chapter 2). It may be accompanied by nausea or headache. One of Dr. Macdonald's patients fainted. Each doctor must, of course, judge the situation of each patient before confronting him with these visual inconsistencies, and the matter of timing can be important, but the new school practitioners are in broad agreement that bringing the patient face to face with his inconsistencies, at some point, is essential to progress in the training program. If they are squarely faced, the patient usually achieves a genuine breakthrough—meaning that his visual perceptions thereafter begin to move more in the direction of reality.

A similar brief trauma or "transition" may occur when, as a result of training, the eyes begin seeing in a different way, but before the body has been able to assimilate the change. This occurs when people suddenly, for the first time in their lives, see the world in the third dimension or achieve a much sharper, brighter sense of color. The body/mind system is temporarily out of synch. The reaction may be exhilaration or depression, but there is always a feeling of disorientation. Dr. Shankman tells his patients that this is a good happening, and that a better matching of their visual and body systems will be the result. He believes that body-awareness training makes the emotional problem of transition easier. Similarly, Dr. Francke believes that good physical conditioning is an essential safeguard against the temporary discomfort of changes in muscles and blood vessels that often take place in the neck and upper back (and ultimately throughout the body) following a visual change. Statistically, new school optometrists do not have serious problems with "critical empathy" or "transition" reactions. Where the training is carefully paced and supervised by the doctor, most patients are affected by only mild and brief disorganizations en route to a visual breakthrough.

POOR TIMING AND COORDINATION

In addition to serious inconsistencies and mismatches there are a number of lesser visual problems whose solution requires improvements in the coordination of the visual system with hand and body movements. The problem may be something as obvious as a child's inability to keep his eyes on a moving target. Or, in tracking such a target, he may jerk his head or his whole body in an excessive effort to control a movement that should be smooth and effortless, indeed without conscious control. When a person must work hard just at the physical act of seeing, it interferes with his *understanding* of what he is seeing. (Dr. Streff compares such a situation to that of a teen-ager learning to drive a car; he is so involved with the mechanics of steering and shifting gears that he just doesn't see what is going on around him.)

Or the problem may be less obvious. It may show up as a subtle difficulty in timing, in being slightly out of step in the coordination between eye and hand. This requires the child to make a small corrective adjustment after each move, which has the effect of disturbing the rhythm of body coordination and of interfering with his ability to interpret what he is seeing. He may lose his place while trying to read, he may reverse letters or words, he may not recognize subtle changes in the meaning of materials being presented. A person with that kind of visual difficulty will find it hard to see precisely how some elements in a situation are similar and how others are different; he may thus fail to see how certain combinations of elements can be made to fit together in a meaningful way. To use a phrase we have encountered earlier, he will have difficulty making accurate relationships.

BODY AWARENESS

Not surprisingly, then, visual-training optometrists use training procedures that test and strengthen a continuous three-step process: the visual system receives stimuli, the mind sends instructions, and the body responds.

Dr. Shankman, for example, has developed two classroom exercises that reflect his belief in the importance of improving body awareness. In the first, the patient walks slowly across the room calling out, and simultaneously executing, such instructions as "right hand up, right hand down, left foot up, left foot down." A variation of the exercise, called Angels in the Snow, is performed with the patient lying face up on the floor. He calls out instructions in a prescribed sequence and moves his arms and legs accordingly—for example, "right arm and right leg out; both arms out, both arms in." These movements are performed to the beat of a metronome —one word for each beat, forty beats per minute.

Dr. Shankman's patients often exhibit an initial inability to match the spoken instruction with the body response— for example, the patient will call out "right hand up" while he is in fact lifting his left hand. Dr. Shankman never corrects the patient for a miscall. His basic instruction is "say what you do and do what you say." He monitors, but insists that the patients evaluate their own performances and correct their own mistakes. In his view, intervention by the doctor would defeat the primary purpose of the exercise, which is to give the patient a firsthand experience in body awareness, synchronization of mind and body, coordination, and control.

Other exercises designed specifically to improve body awareness, balance, and coordination are known as the Ballet, the Balance Rail, and Bilateral Motor Equivalents. These are described in chapter 7. All are based on the assumption that man is a self-directing, self-correcting organism and that vision plays the role of central mediator and coordinator in the body/mind system. Dr. Shankman has found that poor body awareness usually indicates low emotional awareness, but as the former improves, so does the latter. A number of his training patients report that, as they have improved their visual-postural performance, their sex life has improved, too.

Another procedure of similar purpose is known as "standing awareness," which consists of standing comfortably with both eyes closed for periods of ten to thirty minutes. "Kinesthesis" means basically the sensing of when and how the muscles throughout our body are moving. Dr. Skeffington thought the definition should include the sense of "memory of movement," for he believed that a person's habitual posture and observable pattern of body movements are the products of long-term memory lodged in particular muscles, implanted there by the process of repeated instructions and response. Dr. Macdonald believes the standing-awareness procedure is particularly useful "when a major mismatch occurs between the visual and kinesthetic coordinates of the system," for it requires the patient to come to terms with his body posture.

Often the patient does not have an accurate feel for the contours of his body and the space it occupies; for example, he isn't aware that his back is "dented in" or his neck thrust forward; he doesn't sense that his hips or his head are slightly twisted, or that he is carrying more weight on one leg than the other. While the training optometrist—or anyone else looking closely—can see these deficiencies, it is difficult to explain them persuasively to the patient. The value of standing awareness is that it encourages the person to discover these deficiencies for himself, at first hand.

A second purpose of the standing-awareness procedure is to develop a sense of body balance without the help or hindrance of visual reference points. The true centers of balance are the middle of your pelvic area and the middle of your chest; standing awareness teaches you to concentrate on these central points as you stand with both eyes closed. There is a comparable concept in Zen, called centering, which aims at bodily balance and harmony through a concentration of thought and energy in the abdominal area. Concentrating on your "center" will help you to achieve, gradually and over time, a more natural and balanced posture.

Dr. Macdonald claims to have introduced this exercise into

the visual-training program, having derived it from an osteo-path who used it as a basic tool for the diagnosis and self-diagnosis of his patients. He says that "everybody is loaded with torque" and will actually start turning if the normal control mechanisms in the body are sufficiently relaxed as a result of the exercise. What purpose is served? Self-awareness forces the patient to face up to his own mismatches and inconsistencies; and self-diagnosis leads to improvements in the body/mind system via the basic feedback mechanism.

This procedure must be approached with caution and good judgment, and must always be conducted under professional supervision, for it can produce in some patients an emotional reaction. Consistent with Dr. Macdonald's comparison of the visual process with a flow chart in computer technology, every visual problem reflects a limitation of movement or blockage somewhere in the body. As the patient in standing awareness attempts to put his mind in neutral and to "think" through his body alone, being progressively aware of all parts of it and letting it express itself freely in whatever ways seem natural—for example, awareness of a sagging left shoulder, or of discomfort in the lower back—he sometimes vividly recalls happenings in his life that seem somehow related to his postural defects or his visual difficulty. The reaction is complex, related to memory patterns located in particular muscles and conveyed through the central nervous system; if the memories are painful, they may generate strong emotions which are occasionally manifested in weeping, nausea, or depression. As a result, most visual-training practitioners use this procedure for limited periods, especially with children, and they supervise it carefully. They regard it, however, as a technique of great usefulness in enhancing the patient's sense of body awareness.

TAKING IN MORE SPACE

There is an important difference between the new school functionalists and the old school structuralists with regard to the meaning and use of "space," and it is illustrated in the ways the two groups approach the common problem of near-sightedness (myopia).

If you are myopic—shortsighted—most optometrists will prescribe minus lenses (which bring the point of focus closer by compressing the volume of space the eyes can take in). This will improve your sharpness and clarity, but it will also narrow your scope of vision and, as one training optometrist says, has the effect of "bringing the whole world into your lap." Depending on their strength, minus lenses provide the kind of vision you use when you aim a rifle: it is clear and sharp, but narrowly concentrated, and it produces stress for just those reasons. By reducing your field of vision, minus lenses also reduce your capacity to absorb experience visually. By overemphasizing central vision and attenuating peripheral vision, they can adversely affect bodily balance and general coordination, for it is peripheral vision that provides the frame or context for the objects you see; without it, you experience difficulty in precisely locating yourself in space. Thus an attempt to "correct" myopic vision by taking measures that further constrict the field in which the eyes can operate serves chiefly to narrow the general perception, with definite implications for brain activity and personality.

Recognizing this, the new school approach is very different. It tries to reduce myopia, not by bringing about immediate 20/20 acuity, but by training the patient to "see more space," to take in a larger volume of space and more objects within it, through exercises that strengthen the eyes' accommodation to objects both near and far; also by prescribing plus lenses. A plus lens is convex and it gently pushes the point of focus farther away, enabling your eyes to see things in a wider perspective and giving them a cushion of distance that almost always relieves the stress of close work. The new school theory is that the greater the volume of space you can absorb through your eyes, the more information you will have for judging the spatial relationships of objects within your field of vision, and therefore the more accurately and efficiently you will be able to assimilate their meaning and act wisely in your own interest.

New school practitioners acknowledge that, when you first increase your volume intake of space, you may see less clearly than before. But they encourage you to "hold on to the new volume" and work hard at improving your perception of the forms and structure within your enlarged "space world." Acuity will gradually follow. The ultimate objective is to be able to concentrate on one central task, yet be simultaneously aware of all the ramifications and implications surrounding that central point of concentration. In the physical sense, this means broadening your field of vision. In the intellectual sense, it means understanding a widening web of relationships. In both senses, the expansionary result is like a pebble dropped in a pool.

On the other hand, if immediate acuity is held to be the sole or primary goal, and minus lenses are prescribed, you will reduce the volume of space you take in and will thus remain embedded in your old visual-postural set, or indeed become more deeply entrenched. Unlike the structural optometrists, the new school practitioners find nothing fixed about a particular posture, nor anything immutable about myopia. The two are mirror images of each other, reflections of an interlocking balance to which the organism has gravitated in response to the multiple pressures imposed by the particular life of the particular person. Both can be changed, but one cannot be changed without corresponding changes in the other. Teaching the patient to take in a large volume of space is a central element of the new visual training.

Exercises designed to teach the training patient to take in more space and thus enlarge his field of vision include Thumb Pursuits, the Wolff Wand, Pencil and Straw, and Two Sticks. These are described in chapter 7.

THE PERCEPTION OF CONSTANT SIZE

Another reason why the new school places emphasis on the ingestion of "more space" is related to a phenomenon known as the factor of size constancy. People with efficient vision see objects in constant size at varying distances, chiefly because vision is a function of the brain. Descartes, in his famous *Dioptrics,* published in 1637, wrote that when we see objects in space, "it is not the absolute size of the images that counts. Clearly they are a hundred times bigger when the objects are very close to us than when they are ten times farther away, but they do not make us see the objects a hundred times bigger; on the contrary, they seem almost the same size, at any rate so long as we are not deceived by too great a distance."

The point here is that we do not operate by retinal image size alone. If we did, everything close at hand would appear too big and everything far away would appear too small, compared to the realities. What this means is that, through our visual system (the interaction of eyes and brain), we alter the retinal image in accordance with our stored sensory experiences, to create a mental image of what is out there. We then *mentally project* that image out into space and that is what we see. If our visual system is efficient, the size of the image we project will be consistent with the true size of the object—almost regardless of how close or far away the real object is. This is another classic example of the inextricable linkage between the eyes, the brain, and the experience stored in the body/mind system which is retrievable as memory.

Taking in "more space" is important to the achievement of size constancy, for when you take in more space you strengthen your peripheral vision, and it is peripheral vision that provides the frame for what you see with your central vision. It is the strength and efficiency of your peripheral vision that permits you to judge the true size of, and thus the true spatial relationships between, the various objects in the central field. But you cannot have good peripheral vision if your eyes are narrowly channeled and focused close in, nor can you achieve size constancy under such conditions. This is easily demonstrated by a simple procedure. Roll a sheet of paper into a tube and look through it with one eye. You will discover that, as you reduce the diameter of the tube, objects far away get significantly smaller, while near objects assume grotesquely large dimensions. This happens because, as you reduce the diameter of the tube, you reduce the available field of vision and thus your ability to organize what you "see" through your total postural-visual-brain system. You become increasingly dependent on the image size reflected on the retina.

An exercise specifically designed to test and strengthen the perception of size constancy is known as the String Procedure, and is described in chapter 7.

MODELS OF VISUAL PERFORMANCE

The training program conducted by the new school practitioners always starts with a careful assessment of each patient's particular problem, followed by the establishment of at least rough goals toward which the training should be aimed. Dr. Francke favors a "model of optimum visual performance," which is a theoretical model built upon a careful analysis of the patient's visual problem, postural deficiencies, age, energy level, and capacity for undertaking a possibly stressful training program. It includes a judgment as to whether the patient has a visual deficiency in urgent need of correction, or has only a moderate problem, or is seeking primarily to enhance an already excellent performance. Dr. Robert Kraskin develops training goals related to specific objectives in the patient's life—for example, to play a better game of golf, to read for three hours without fatigue, to see the opera stage clearly from a seat in the balcony. Dr. Shankman believes that long-range goals are important, but that the patient usually places more weight on short-term tangible progress. He has found it is progress that motivates his patients and makes them eager for more training.

Whether simple or elaborate, formal or implicit, such goals and models do help to guide and measure a process that is inherently too complicated to be fully or directly observed. Indeed, when the patient is in visual training, performing a variety of body-awareness, balancing, and eye exercises over

a period of weeks and months, the complexities of the interactions between his eyes, his brain, and the muscular and
nervous systems throughout his body are almost surely beyond
full comprehension by anyone—even the best-trained and
most astute optometrists or ophthalmologists. They can observe changes in visual performance, and can take from them
clues as to which procedures they should reinforce, which
they should curtail, and whether a given pace of training is
appropriate in the circumstances. But they cannot pretend
to understand exactly how these changes in the organism are
actually taking place. That remains one of Nature's secrets.

Dr. Francke made an assessment of me (Townsend Hoopes)
at the time I was considering becoming a training patient, in
the late summer of 1975. Even before I got to his office, he
had gained the impression that I was a somewhat "overworked
person" because I had "changed or canceled five appoint-
ments at the last minute." When I finally arrived for an
interview, his first impressions were these: "(a) the patient
looked fatigued; (b) slumped posture generally, with a leftward tilt to the shoulders and also a head tilt; (c) walked as
though the upper part of his body had nothing to do with
the lower part; (d) heavy lower body; (e) heavily muscled
overall; (f) obviously he was exerting a great deal of energy
to handle his body; (g) asked good questions."

The 21-point eye examination that he conducted a week
later revealed "a very stressful type of vision, complicated
by a vertical phoria in right eye; his unaided acuity at distance is poor enough to cause stress, and so is his corrected
acuity at near." It also showed that "the patient pours a great
deal of energy into seeing at both far and near; measures of
reserve energy are low; there is a definite tilt in his visual
performance consistent with his body tilt." The basic con-

clusion was that "the patient is going all out" to achieve reasonable binocular efficiency. From this analysis, Dr. Francke developed a set of general goals for my training program. They aimed at achieving: (a) a significant reduction of visual stress at both near point and distance; (b) improved acuity at both near point and distance; (c) an elimination of the postural slump and the leftward tilt; (d) some weight reduction, particularly in the lower body; and (e) more energy.

To move me toward this "model of improved visual performance," the doctor first gave me low plus reading glasses with a much larger lens area. I had been wearing half-glasses for reading, which rather constricted the area of intake, and the mere fact that the new glasses allowed me to cover a wider field made seeing and reading immediately easier. He then designed a training program aimed primarily at relieving the stress in my system while moving gradually to strengthen my distance vision. The elements included: (a) body-awareness and balancing exercises to create a greater "physical looseness" and to improve my "gross balancing ability"; (b) walking and jogging several times a week to break down the "artificial barriers" between my upper and lower body and to move me toward a more harmonious visual-postural alignment; (c) simple eye exercises at home to strengthen my ability to shift smoothly from near focus to far focus and vice versa; (d) eye exercises with "doubling glasses" and other training lenses, to be performed in the classroom under supervision; and (e) performing all of these activities at a reasonable pace so as to avoid a "transition" reaction severe enough to take me away from my job for even a few days.

My compliance with the program fell short of the doctor's expectations. Originally, I was diligent about classroom training, but neglectful of the exercises assigned for performance at home; later I became religious about home training, but delinquent about attending the classroom. And with regard to physical conditioning, while I jogged, swam, performed calisthenics, and played tennis, all with regularity and zest, I did not walk far enough or often enough to please my doctor. Despite these backslidings, examinations about ten months after the training started, and again six months later, showed encouraging progress. I made relatively small, though respectable, improvements in my distance vision (from 20/60 to 20/50 in one eye, and from 20/60 to 20/40 in the other), but I did achieve a nearly 80 percent reduction in the vertical phoria.

Most important, I experienced steady improvements in my day-to-day performance in the real world, improvements that the doctor regarded as disproportionate both to my "input" effort and to my optometric changes. My eyestrain was virtually gone; as a direct result, I had the sense of enjoying a measurably higher energy level than ever before, even when I had been a good deal younger. I continued to commute frequently between offices in Washington and New York, handling a wide range of legislative, legal, and administrative problems directly and through a sizable staff, and traveled more widely on related business—to London, Tokyo, Frankfurt, Moscow, Jerusalem, Montreal, and San Francisco in 1976 and 1977 alone. My training lasted about fifteen months. As a result, I am certain that I now handle my life and work with higher energy, greater efficiency, and less fatigue than was previously the case.

The amazing truth is that, when the body/mind system achieves better internal balance and greater flexibility of response, it is able to synthesize all information more easily and coherently, making for a more efficient performance overall and creating a feeling of harmony and well-being. The new level of performance is sustainable when it has become biologically the most comfortable and economical performance for the body/mind system. Such are the wonderful fruits of effective visual training.

Once the new level of performance can be sustained, the optometrist and the patient should decide whether this improvement is sufficient, or whether the training should be continued with the aim of attaining an even higher level of visual performance. It is a decision that should be carefully weighed in each case, and (where time and money are not severe constraints) we would counsel patients to be ambitious for themselves, rather than being satisfied with a modest improvement. For the visual system is capable of very considerable improvement, always influenced by variables—including physical health, lifestyle, and emotional state. Some of these are, of course, never fully controllable, but it is surprising how many of them can be effectively managed and influenced within the framework of a devoted and disciplined effort. The case histories we have used in this book testify to that truth. If you have the motivation and discipline to take yourself in hand—to eat, drink, work, and exercise in ways that do not abuse your body and mind—you can readily establish the physical preconditions, the "personal environment" in which a well-defined and conscientiously pursued program of visual training can produce steady, even dramatic improvement over a period of weeks and months. While the possibilities for continuing progress are not, of course, totally open-ended, they are much higher and wider than people unacquainted with the new visual training can appreciate.

Nor is age a fundamental obstacle to improvement. No claim is made, of course, that the new visual training can reverse the aging process, but the adverse effects of age on visual performance can be slowed through a carefully designed training program, not so much by improving the eyes per se as by reducing the wear and tear of stress, which tends to become progressive in older people and which is, of course, the primary cause of aging. Diet and exercise are also vital factors in relieving stress and extending the years of active pleasurable life, as we shall try to make clear in chapter 9.

Seven

Training Exercises

THE LEADING PRACTITIONERS of the new school sometimes differ from one another on particular visual-training techniques, but they are fully agreed on the fundamental purposes of training. They are agreed also that this involves considerations much broader than merely training the eye. Procedures designed to exercise the muscles of the eye can produce temporary changes in eyesight, but, as Dr. Shankman has expressed it, "to get permanent improvement, you must achieve true vision changes, meaning changes in mind/eye synchronization, in time/space matching, in coordination of the whole body/mind system. Such visual changes are brought about by a combination of diet, physical conditioning, improved body awareness, and eye exercises. It is a comprehensive self-monitoring process." When this process is successful, it "builds in" the visual improvements.

The training exercises described and explained in this chapter are designed, collectively, to produce "true vision changes" and to "build in" the improvements. They are simple, interesting, and involve little or no equipment and no lenses. They are activities in what professionals call "real space/time," as opposed to the "restructured space/time" which is created by bending radiant energy with lenses, prisms, and mirrors. Accordingly, you can try them without any appreciable risk and quite possibly with measurable benefit. But it should be clear from the line of reasoning in this chapter, and indeed throughout this book, that full benefits can be realized only within the context of a visual-training program prescribed for you personally by a professional optometrist who has examined your eyes and diagnosed your problem, and who provides periodic supervision and assessment.

The optometrist's role is decisive. At the same time, as has been noted, the training is largely a biofeedback process involving self-monitoring and self-correcting by the patient, and Dr. Macdonald has said plainly that "the patient will do the correcting, not the optometrist." Through his experience, the optometrist will provide directional guides which will enable the patient to monitor his own visual process. The patient will thereby discover the consistencies and mismatches inherent in his personal style of processing visual information, but what he does with this new insight will be largely up to him. The optometrist serves as the indispensable coach, but "the patient will decide to change or not to change his visual habits."

Some new school practitioners practice "sequential" and some practice "directional" training. Dr. Shankman usually assigns three basic procedures to beginning patients, and then adds two more after three to five weeks. Dr. Francke assigns a patient only one procedure at a time. As he has put it, "these are not sequential procedures, they are directional procedures. The essence of directional training is that you can only give the first set of instructions to a patient and then you have to watch and see what the patient does, and then you can give him the second set, and the second set will be different for everyone, and in fact the first set is generally different for everyone."

Dr. Macdonald, who prefers a step-by-step approach, uses cassette tapes to guide the home training of some of his patients, and he finds that "it is amazing the complexity of subject matter that can be sent home with a willing patient." He uses cassettes to introduce the patient to new training techniques, and uses the classroom visits to practice and refine the exercises begun at home. "When the program is working ideally, the patients come to the optometrist with questions that have been suggested while practicing."

The following training exercises are widely used by new school practitioners. Their descriptions in this chapter are grouped according to the major element or purpose of the program they are designed to serve.

BODY-AWARENESS PROCEDURES

The following exercises, designed to improve body awareness, balance, and coordination, are known as the Ballet, the Balance Rail, and Bilateral Motor Equivalents.

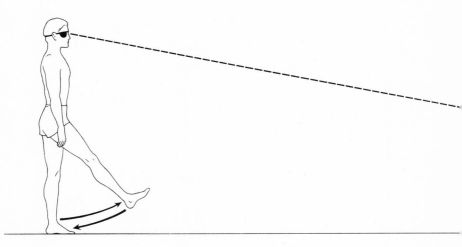

1. The Ballet Exercise

A simple exercise to increase body awareness, balance, flexibility, and control is called the Ballet Exercise. It is done by covering one eye with an eye patch. In bare or stocking feet, you stand in a comfortable posture, directing your line of sight to a point twenty or thirty feet in front of you. Holding that target, you slowly raise your left leg in front of you, as high and as straight as possible. Then you slowly lower it, but without letting the foot touch the ground; then raise it in the same fashion to the side and lower it, again without allowing the foot to touch the ground. Then you raise the leg behind you and slowly return it to the ground. Next repeat the exercise with the right leg. You then shift the eye patch to the other eye and perform the procedure with first the left and then the right leg (see illustration). Finally, you perform the exercise with both eyes covered or closed.

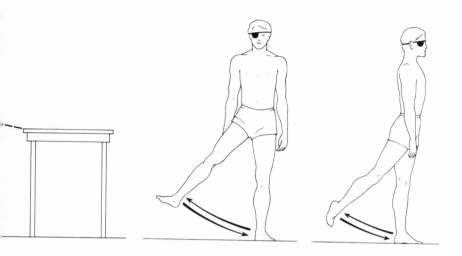

Initially most people discover they have far less control of their bodies than they had thought, and have particular trouble visualizing the room and the position of their bodies in it when both eyes are covered. There is special difficulty in visualizing the area behind you.

Like standing awareness, the Ballet is designed to strengthen your sense of bodily awareness and control, and your sense of spatial orientation, by teaching you to concentrate on the two primary centers of gravity—the pelvic area and the middle of the chest. Binocular mismatches cannot be corrected by simply concentrating harder with the eyes. It requires, first, the achievement of a better balance and alignment throughout the body/mind system. Body awareness is the basis of body control; better body control is in turn the key to improved posture, and both are essential to improve the efficiency with which your visual system processes information—that is, achieves a more accurate matching of visual perception with the true characteristics of objects in the physical world. As Dr. Francke has put it: "If we wish to improve our visual performance, we must alter the way we use our body by moving it toward a balanced, ideal position. . . . This balanced posture implies balancing our bodies in all dimensions."

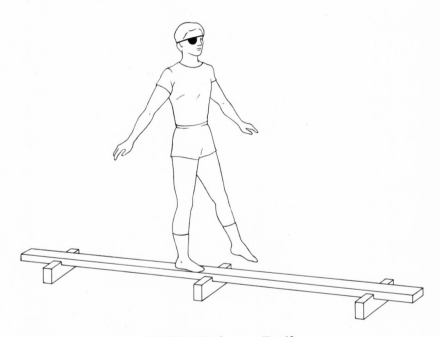

2. The Balance Rail

New school optometrists tell the story of their mentor, Dr. A. M. Skeffington, the pioneer visual-training expert, who was waiting for his train at the railroad station of a small midwestern town many years ago. For diversion he started walking on one of the railroad tracks to see if he could balance himself. After a while he came upon a young girl doing the same thing, indeed approaching him on the same rail. They looked each other straight in the eye and continued forward. Just before they met, both stepped off the track to allow the other to pass. As the girl stepped off, Dr. Skeffington noted that she went "from straight-eyed to strabismic"— that is, to cross-eyed. From this he deduced that she was normally cross-eyed, but that when she was forced to maintain bodily balance on the rail, her eyes had temporarily straightened out. This observation strengthened Dr. Skeffington's view that the eye is malleable and that good visual performance depends upon the achievement of a harmonious alignment between eyes and body. His judgment led to the widespread use of the four-inch Balance Rail (mounted a few inches off the ground) as a basic device in optometric visual training.

You walk on the Balance Rail in stocking feet with one eye patched and the other eye seeking to take in as much space *and as many objects as possible*. You quickly discover that holding in view multiple reference points, simultaneously, gives you a much more stable balance than if you fix your eye on only one point. For just as in aiming an artillery piece by triangulation, or in fixing the position of a ship by reference to several stars or terrain features on the horizon, you locate your body more accurately and precisely by reference to several objects in your field of vision than by reference to only one of them. You walk both forward *and backward* on the Balance Rail. And when you have mastered it with first one and then the other eye covered, you seek to master it with both eyes covered. The key to success in this last variation is to visualize the reference points in the room as you remember them, but to concentrate mainly on "centering" your balance in your abdomen and lower chest.

The Balance Rail is used in thousands of regular and special educational schools; sometimes a tilted board is used.

Herman A. Witkin has described experiments designed to determine an individual's perception of the true vertical. One of these employs a small room (like a stage set) mounted on a machine which permits the room to be tilted to any degree to the left or right, as well as a chair for the patient which can similarly be tilted independently of the stage-set room. The interior design of the set provides many clearly defined lines that accentuate its vertical and horizontal axes. With the room and chair tilted at the same angle, the experimenter moves the chair at the patient's direction until the patient reports himself to be upright. Witkin found that those people who depend exclusively or primarily on visual reference for their sense of the vertical often believed they were sitting upright when the chair was tilted as much as 35 degrees. Conversely, people who were more sensitive to the inner balance of their bodies had no trouble in sensing when they were tilted to the left or right, regardless of the angle of the visual reference points. (When the patient closed his eyes, he could of course immediately adjust to the true vertical even if he were a person who relied primarily upon visual references. This ability to adjust is a function of the vestibular components—the semicircular canals and otolith structures in the ears.) You can test your own sense of the vertical by trying to judge the attitude of an airliner in which you are a passenger when it is flying through clouds or darkness. More sensitive people can tell whether it is banking or climbing, even without visual clues.

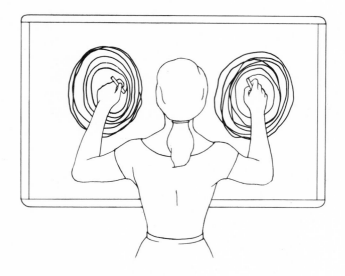

3. Bilateral Motor Equivalents

The set of exercises known as Bilateral Motor Equivalents is designed to balance out the various coordinating mechanisms by reducing the pronounced tendency in each of us to left or right "sidedness." The body being an interacting complex of subsystems mediated by vision and the brain, each bodily movement is normally directed by or through the dominant "side," but each movement always involves a counterbalancing movement executed by the other or nonpreferred "side." In each case, the quality of the total performance is limited by the relative inefficiency of the counterbalancing movement —and that movement is usually weak or awkward because we have done nothing to develop strength or agility on the nonpreferred side. Dr. Harmon, who understood this prob-

113

lem, devised a series of exercises in which the patient draws large circles on a chalkboard, first with the dominant hand, then with the nonpreferred hand, and then with both hands simultaneously in a variety of clockwise and counterclockwise movements. Using the same principle, others have moved the exercises off the chalkboard and out into the real world by instructing their patients to carry out a number of ordinary tasks—for example, buttoning their shirts, shaving, eating, and dialing a telephone—all with the "wrong," or nonpreferred, hand. Diligent practice leads to a far more even-handed dexterity, with important implications for a better balance and coordination of the whole body/mind system.

TAKING IN MORE SPACE

The following exercises, designed to teach the training patient to take in more space and thus enlarge his field of vision, are known as Thumb Pursuits, the Wolff Wand, Two Sticks, and Pencil and Straw.

4. Thumb Pursuits

A widely used eye-training exercise is a deceptively simple procedure called Thumb Pursuits. It consists of standing erect, covering one eye with an eye patch, and then following the upright thumb of your right hand with your right eye (or of your left hand with your left eye) as the thumb is moved slowly in a random pattern, in and out, up, down, and around. This exercise has several different aims, but the most basic is to see the thumb while simultaneously extending your eye's coverage to as many other objects and as much space in the room as possible. The idea is to achieve a clear focus on the thumb in the near distance and *at the same time* a clear focus on other objects farther away.

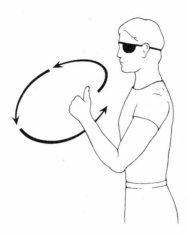

As you perform the exercise, you should ask yourself the following questions:

1. Can you see the thumb clearly at all positions within the reach of your arm? If not, at what positions and distances is it blurred?
2. When the thumb is clear and sharp, is the rest of the room also in focus, or is it blurred?
3. If you move your posture toward the ideal upright balanced position, does this help to keep both the thumb and the rest of the room in simultaneous focus?
4. Conversely, if you deliberately slump, how does that affect your ability to focus?
5. How much volume of space can you take in at one time? If you seek to maximize the volume, how does this

affect the acuity with which you see the thumb or other specific objects?

6. How can you improve acuity in the central area without losing volume?

7. How can you improve acuity in the left and right peripheries without losing volume?

8. Does your thumb vary in size as you move it in and out, or does it remain constant? Do you see any advantage in having it remain a constant size?

The way in which you answer these questions begins to define your present visual performance, meaning the volume of space you can ingest and the control you can impose on that volume under varying conditions of distance, focal point of attention, and posture. At the beginning, most patients are unable to achieve a simultaneous clarity of their thumb and the background objects; most will lose acuity of the thumb if they stretch their eye to take in a greater volume of space; most will have only limited peripheral vision; most will see their thumb grow bigger or smaller as it moves closer or farther away from the eye. The exercise is thus a useful introduction to the truth that the moving thumb exists not in isolation, but within a three-dimensional world comprising you, your total field of vision, and all other objects within that field. How well you organize that total volume of space will determine how clearly you see the thumb; the more reference points you can see clearly, the more accurately you will fix the thumb target in space.

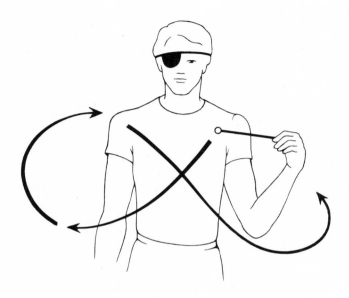

5. The Wolff Wand

A variation of the Thumb Pursuit exercise is the Wolff Wand (named for its inventor, Dr. Bruce Wolff of Cii. cinnati), in which a small steel ball-bearing mounted on a metal wand is similarly manipulated, by either the patient or the doctor. This is an exercise particularly well adapted to stretching and thus strengthening peripheral vision, since the wand can be moved to either side as far as the arm extends (and should normally be moved in an irregular pattern, both back and forth and at varying distances from the eyes; see illustration). It is important to see peripheral objects clearly, rather than merely being aware of their existence, for they provide the frame of the picture and thus give clarity to the objects in your central field of vision. The clarity of the central target is proportionate to the clarity of the peripheral field.

The basic objective of both the Thumb Pursuit and the Wolff Wand tracking procedure is to teach you to follow a target smoothly and easily with the eye, and to know where the target is in space. Because the target is continually changing its location (often on all three planes simultaneously), you are constantly required to make different spatial calculations in a three-dimensional world. This involves you in what new school optometrists call "accommodative rock," which has nothing to do with modern music but refers to the eye's ability to shift smoothly from near to far focus and vice versa. These exercises, like a number of others, also teach you that your own body is the center and basic frame of reference for all of your judgments about objects in your field of vision. *What* you see depends not only on *where,* but also on *how* you stand.

As we established in chapter 6, learning to ingest a greater volume of space is a fundamental object of the training. For the more space volume you can take in, the more accurately you can see the objects in spatial relationship one to the other. And the more clearly you can distinguish those objects (their different shapes and textures), the better you can interpret and utilize the visual information they impart.

As Dr. Gesell has explained, the major elements of the visual process fall into a three-step sequence: (1) the visual system seeks and holds an image; (2) it discriminates and defines the image; and (3) it interprets the image through the experience and memory stored in the brain. The original perception of the image thus leads to ascending degrees of attention, identification, and interpretation (or mental synthesis). It is in the last step that vision performs its sophisticated fusion with the brain, as we showed in chapter 4.

Therefore, the higher the level of your visual performance, the greater physical and mental efficiency you will achieve— you will read better, think faster, or prove more expert at setting up plays during the course of a fast-moving basketball game.

The practical advantages of being able to take in a larger volume of space and to be aware of the precise location of objects within it are evident in the basic matters of reading and driving. Reading depends on the information you can grasp in each ocular fixation. As each fixation takes about one fifth of a second, you have about five fixations per second. How much volume you see in that time determines what you can supply to your brain in order to get meaning from a printed page. Accordingly, if your perceived volume within each fixation includes a whole phrase, a whole sentence, or several sentences, you will be a more efficient reader than the person who can absorb, within each fixation, only a word or two. The same argument applies with even greater force to the business of driving a car, for that is a survival process. Frequently, one new school practitioner has observed, "our lives literally depend on how much information we can get in one or two fixations." But volume alone is obviously not a decisive advantage. It does you no good to see a large area of the printed page if the acuity (quality) level is too low for you to identify the words quickly and without strain. Similarly, an ability to see the horizon beyond the highway will not help if you cannot identify the moving vehicles in your immediate vicinity and what they are doing. To be useful, the ability to take in a larger volume must be accompanied by a high level of accuracy.

Greater volume *with* acuity is thus a basic aim of the training, and procedures like Thumb Pursuits and the Wolff Wand can assist in its realization.

119

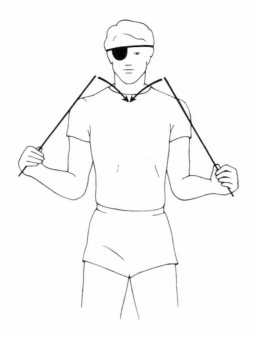

6. Two Sticks

Another excellent exercise involves two round sticks or dowels, each about twenty-four inches long, one held in each hand. With one eye covered, you bring the sticks together from various distances and various angles (see illustration). The purpose is to test how much space you can "control" in terms of accurate depth perception horizontally, vertically, and diagonally. Standing erect, you hold the sticks so that one is extended farther than the other and their tips are several inches apart. You next determine the specific point in space where you believe the tips of the sticks will touch if moved toward each other. You then move both sticks quickly to that point. In the beginning you will miss rather frequently, even from a distance of only a few inches. One stick will be higher or lower, and the two ends will pass in space instead of touching. If you miss, it means you have not sufficiently organized your field of vision—by fixing the central objects in relation to objects in the background and on the peripheries; or it means your hand-eye coordination is faulty. It may reflect deficiencies in both of these matters. *You should note that not only space but also space/time is involved in this exercise.*

You should immediately correct the error by bringing the stick ends together, and then repeat the exercise from the same distance several times—as many times as are required to perfect your depth perception and your eye-hand coordination at that distance. Next do the same thing with the other eye patched. Then widen the starting distance between the sticks and vary the angle of approach. And do it again. It is an exercise of wide variations and great training value.

7. Pencil and Straw

A variant of the Two Sticks exercise involves a pencil and a hollow drinking straw. Tape the straw, horizontally at the center, to any free-standing vertical that will permit a clear approach from either side. Then, with one eye covered, hold the pencil in the left hand some twelve to eighteen inches from the left end of the straw (or in the right hand the same distance from the right end). The object is to line up the pencil and the straw, perceiving them as a single horizontal line and judging for depth perception. You then move the pencil in a single swift motion in an effort to run the pencil tip inside the straw (see illustration, page 122). As in the Two Sticks exercise, you will probably miss frequently in the be-

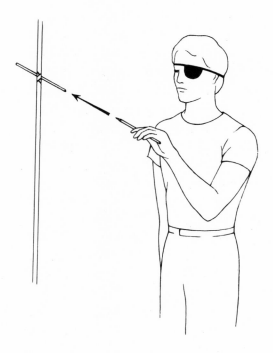

ginning, moving the pencil slightly above or below the straw, or slightly behind or in front of it. Correct each error immediately, and repeat until you have achieved perfect eye-hand control of this space/time relationship.

SIZE CONSTANCY

The following exercise, designed to test and strengthen the perception of size constancy, is known as the String Procedure.

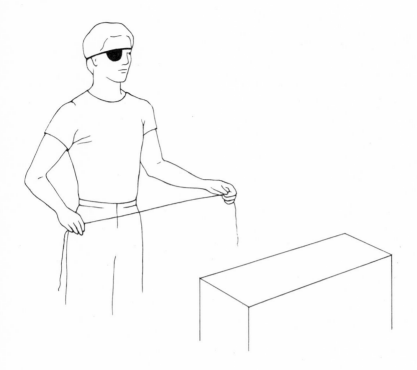

8. The String Procedure

The accurate sensing of the size of a particular object at varying distances in space is not an easy or automatic achievement. But, as we established in chapter 6, the perception of constant size is an important measure of visual efficiency. It depends, first of all, on your knowing how much space the object occupies; it also depends on an ability to organize your field of vision—to see all the objects within it, including those on both peripheries, and to judge accurately the distances between each of them and the central target object, as well as the distance of each of the objects from you. The

String Procedure illustrates this problem and challenge. With one eye covered, you stand in the center of the room holding a piece of string four or five feet long outstretched between your hands. You look around and pick any measurement of distance you think is within the span of your outstretched arms—for example, the width of a bureau. You then ask yourself how far apart you have to hold your hands to make the distance between them agree exactly with the width of the bureau. You then adjust your hands on the string and move to the bureau to see if your estimate is correct (see illustration). Most people fail this test initially; if you pass it, you already have a reasonably good sense of size constancy.

But the harder part of the exercise comes next. You correct the length of string to match the width of the bureau. You then back away slowly, trying simultaneously to maintain a visual match between the bureau and the string. You try to see how far you can back away before the string no longer appears to match the width of the bureau. At that point, you should stop, take a deep breath, and begin to apply the fundamentals of visual training. In essence, the problem is to organize your field of vision: (a) assume an erect posture, as close as possible to the ideal; (b) take in as much volume of space as possible in the room, being sharply aware of objects on the periphery and judging their distance from each other and from the bureau; and (c) determine how much volume each of the peripheral objects occupies (this involves a judgment as to the true size of each). This exercise takes practice and more practice, as well as considerable tears and sweat. It cannot be mastered immediately. Gradually, however, you will discover that, as you become more aware of the precise information contained in your field of vision, your sense of size constancy will improve.

VARIABLE-PURPOSE EXERCISE

A variable exercise using a rubber ball suspended from the ceiling by a string is helpful in improving the patient's visual skills in several different areas. This is known as the Marsden Ball Technique.

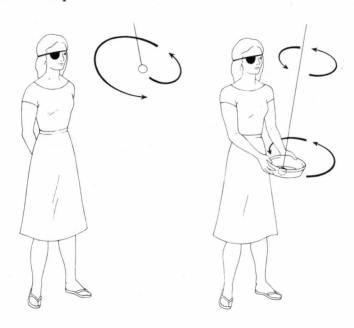

9. The Marsden Ball Technique

The Marsden Ball Technique (invented by Dr. Carl D. Marsden of Rocky Ford, Colorado, about twenty-seven years ago) starts by suspending a rubber ball from the ceiling at a height between the chest and chin. As originally used, the ball was swung in a circle or an arc, and the patient followed it with both eyes open or with one eye covered. It was, in short, a simple pursuit procedure designed to require the muscles of the eye to lengthen and contract as the distance between the eye and the ball was lengthened and shortened. As with the Wolff Wand and Thumb Pursuits, the purpose of this exercise was to develop "accommodative rock," meaning the ability of the eye to shift smoothly from near to far focus and vice versa. But the Marsden Ball Technique has undergone considerable development and refinement over the years, and now frequently encompasses a whole series of procedures that advance progressively in difficulty and sophistication:

- In one variation, letters of the alphabet are pasted on the ball, and you are instructed to call out the letters you see as the ball moves through its circle or arc.
- In another variation, you hold a pencil poised like a dart beside your ear; you then attempt, in a swift thrust, to hit the moving ball at various positions on the arc.
- Not only to test eye-hand coordination but to engage the whole body in rhythmic movement in relation to the moving ball, some practitioners have introduced a basket, three or four inches deep and about the size of a small salad bowl. You hold the basket in both hands and move it beneath the moving ball, endeavoring to keep the ball *inside of but not touching* the basket; as the ball swings in its circle, your whole body moves rhythmically with it, except for your feet, which remain comfortably planted. You look like someone doing a stationary waltz; you are in fact exercising and refining the motor control that is the basis of superior eye-body coordination.

Eight

Lens Training

OPTOMETRY'S UNIQUENESS lies in its ability to use lenses. They are the most potent visual-training tool, and they set the pace of training, requiring the patient to use his visual system more intensively and to adjust it more finely than does any other type of procedure. Lenses are the most efficient way to help the visual process to improve the visual process, and they should be used in every case of visual training. Lenses alter the way the patient sees the world, yet this altered perception still allows him to receive all of the original visual information. Because the visual system is the master coordinator of the body/mind system, the act of altering perception through the use of lenses forces adjustments in posture, in coordination, and indeed in all bodily and mental functions affected by the central and autonomic nervous systems.

Lenses thus possess dramatic power and are usually the decisive element in visual training. They must be carefully prescribed and adjusted at various stages of the training to be certain they are moving the patient in the desired direction, without undue stress. The power and importance of lenses are the principal reasons why visual training cannot be a do-it-yourself program, but requires the initial diagnosis and the continuing guidance of a professional optometrist.

This chapter endeavors to demonstrate the power and importance of lenses in visual training by describing the new school use of a particular kind of lens to correct the widespread condition of myopia (nearsightedness).

MYOPIA AND THE PLUS LENS

Functional optometry has discovered several fascinating truths about the physical aspects of reading and thinking, all of which reinforce the central belief of the new school that physical space/time images seen in your field of vision are the building blocks of your reasoning power.

Vision, like speech and thought, is a symbolizing process— we label an object with a word. When you read the word "cow," your mind leaps away from the page to your image of the animal (memory is triggered by symbols). When you do so, tests show that you actually focus *through* and beyond the page to visualize the cow. By way of contrast, people who read literally—that is, who simply call out each word without understanding it—focus on the actual word and the page. They are locked into the here and now of real time. But success in schoolwork or in any other intellectual pursuit requires what Dr. Streff calls "the flexibility of eye and visual skills literally to see in two places at one time"; it requires the ability simultaneously to *see* the language code and to *translate* it into meaningful terms, and tests show that this requires a highly developed ability to control the focus of the eyes, to shift quickly and easily back and forth between the short focus on the word itself and the longer focus on the idea and meaning beyond the word. Beginners and students with learning difficulties cannot do this efficiently. But an able student can read aloud with smoothness and comprehension, his eyes running ahead of his voice to see and understand the next word or phrase, holding on to two different images at one time without losing his place. Dr. Macdonald calls this skill "accommodative lag."

This evidence of how the visual system progresses from literal perception to comprehension, and of how progress depends on increasing the flexibility and precision control of the eye movements, bears directly on the interesting cause-and-effect relationship between intense close work and myopia. As we have seen, beginning readers focus on the words and phrases. This involves taking in literal stimuli, but not visualizing their meaning. In order to get beyond literalness to comprehension of the symbols, students and scholars must push the focus of the eye through the word and through and beyond the page. When this process is pursued intensively and over a long period of time, it leads to myopia. Why? Because the struggle to comprehend—to translate word symbols into genuine meaning—causes the visual system to close in, to focus more sharply on the central object, as in the act of aiming a rifle. When this occurs, the system tends to go rigid. The eye focus gets narrow and fixed, the neck and the back get stiff. Both peripheral and distance vision are sacrificed in the effort to focus all available energy on the complicated problem of mastering the intellectual symbols. As we said earlier, myopia is a widespread phenomenon in our paper-oriented, white-collar society, but sustained close work of any kind (from sewing to making jewelry) also leads to myopia, and for the same reason—because it requires a narrow intensity of focus.

In 1959, Dr. Darrell Boyd Harmon demonstrated, in the course of a seminar in Cincinnati, that the application of a simple plus lens can reduce the physiological stress that is present throughout the body/mind system when a person is engaged in "problem solving" involving the eyes and the brain. This gave scientific verification to a truth that had been evident from clinical practice for a number of years. Since then, the plus lens has become a special tool of functional optometry, used not only to give immediate relief from acute visual stress, but also to provide protection against myopia for persons whose jobs involve a large volume of close or analytical reading. A plus lens, being convex, spreads the energy transmitted from the light source across a wider area of the retina. This aids the effort to take in more space; it also strengthens peripheral vision and so facilitates the making of accurate relationships.

Dr. Streff emphasizes his view that visual-training patients who have improved their vision need the protection of plus lenses. "As you improve a patient's visual coordination, you need to provide plus lenses for near work, in order to permit him to sustain his new near-point efficiency without constricting into myopia. For as the patient processes more information (as a result of greater efficiency through visual training), there is a strong tendency to close in, in order to get magnification. Plus lenses permit the patient to continue a high volume of efficient processing without going into the constriction of myopia."

The following brief case histories illustrate the important role of plus lenses in the new functional optometry.

Julia

Julia underwent eye surgery in 1975 when she was 8 years old. The operation was for the resection of the left inferior oblique muscle (the muscle responsible for elevating the eye and turning it in). As a result of the surgery, Julia tilted her head at an extreme angle, virtually laying it against her left shoulder. This condition persisted for four years until her parents, in despair, brought her to a visual training optometrist when she was 12.

The optometrist found that the basic problem was a severe "alternating hypertropia"—an uncontrollable tendency of first one eye and then the other to gaze upward at a sharp angle. The right eye was worse than the left, but both eyes tended to jump up and down in the course of reading. Julia instinctively tilted her head to eliminate the effort required to lower the right eye; with the head tilted, she didn't have to pull it down, but could gaze more or less horizontally at the target. She was also nearsighted (myopic). She held her head in her left hand while reading; she read slowly and with low comprehension and short attention span. Although she was already in a special class for slow learners, she remained nervous, irritable, inattentive, and obviously stressed. She read primarily with her right eye.

The doctor used training lenses to teach each of Julia's eyes, separately, to focus accurately on an object at various distances, since the basic problem was that each eye tended to see a given object at a different distance. To avoid the confusion caused by this inaccurate processing of information, Julia unconsciously blocked out one eye most of the time.

During the first three months of visual training, there was no change in Julia's condition. Then one day she saw both eyes in a mirror at a distance of six feet using a training device called "polaroid lenses"; this indicated she was now using both eyes, rather than suppressing her left eye. At four months, she began to hold her head erect while reading. After five months she had virtually eliminated the tilt and was doing homework without apparent strain. The hypertropia at far distances was gone; the eyes retained a *tendency* to flip up, but Julia could now control this by muscular exertion.

After six months, the doctor prescribed bifocals (a plus 75 lens for near work, but just plain glass for distance) to ease the nearsightedness. When a person is being brought out of myopia through visual training, she needs a plus lens to support her new ability to converge her eyes at a greater distance. The need for plus lens reading glasses is thus a sign of progress and improvement.

By the seventh month of training, Julia's reading and writing had greatly improved. During the ninth month she began to ride a two-wheel bicycle, which had been quite impossible for her when her head was tilted; this meant she had now achieved a much better balance of her whole body/mind system. After the twelfth month, she was a well-organized child, showing good physical coordination and able to play fast-moving games. She was less and less dependent on her lenses. The doctor felt Julia was approaching the "stabilization phase" which signals the logical completion of visual training.

Helen

Helen was a college student. She had worn contact lenses for seven years without any change in prescription, and went to a visual-training optometrist in 1975 because she was suffering from severe tension in her eyes, her forehead, and the bridge of her nose. The tension produced frequent headaches. She also felt she was "overfocusing"—meaning that she saw too much detail close in, but nothing much beyond five feet—and she sensed this was producing not only a visual but also a psychological and intellectual restriction.

The training optometrist gave her a set of plus glasses (.50 diopter) to wear over the contact lenses, which reduced the net lens power from -3.75 to -3.25. This immediately reduced the tension, enlarged her field of vision, and soon caused a shift to a more comfortable visual-postural balance. Over the next eleven months, he made progressive changes in both the contact lenses and the glasses, gradually reducing the net lens power by nearly 80 percent, as shown in the following chart:

Date	Contact Lens	Glasses	Net Lens Power
8/27/75	-3.75		-3.75
1/30/76	-3.25	$+0.50$	-2.75
3/13/76	-2.75	$+0.75$	-2.00
6/25/76	-2.75	$+1.25$	-1.50
9/3/76	-2.50	$+1.50$	-1.00

As a result of wearing lenses that induced her to take in a greater volume of space, Helen lost her tension and her headaches. She achieved a broader visual and also a broader psychological perspective, learned to read faster and with better comprehension, and found her college studies easier to grasp and complete. "I write with greater facility now, and can actually 'see' how sentences should be constructed."

Nine

Diet and Exercise

AS WE SOUGHT to establish in the first chapter of this book, and as discussion in all of the subsequent chapters should have made clear, the new school takes not only a functional but also a holistic approach to vision and its ramifications. In the context of visual training, a holistic approach means a belief that a specific defect within the body/mind system is not correctable by an exclusive attack on that defect, but rather by taking a range of measures to restore the harmonious functioning, coordination, balance, and efficiency of the system as a whole. As the previous chapters have sought to show, there is the most intimate linkage between vision and the brain, vision and posture, vision and coordination. The several case histories have demonstrated that disorders ranging from hypertension and backache to menstrual irregularities are often caused by eyes that coordinate badly with each other or that are otherwise not in harmonious alignment with other components of the body/mind system; they have also shown, conversely, that postural deviations and prolonged physical or mental strain can cause badly coordinated eyes. In short, the determining factor for the health of the body/mind system is not the condition of any single component element, but rather the condition of the whole.

Diet is increasingly recognized as a factor of fundamental influence in the health of the human body/mind system, even though it continues to be mindlessly discounted by the upper and older reaches of the conventional medical profession. There is still a surprisingly widespread failure to see that a bad diet is a health-destroying living habit, working steadily to impair chemical and metabolic order and to weaken the system's resistance to harmful bacteria. Similarly, they fail to see a good diet as a truly vital factor in maintaining the strength, balance, energy, and efficiency of the system, and thus in safeguarding it against the derangements that constitute poor health and serious illness. Thomas A. Edison, who, in addition to inventing the electric light bulb, gave much wise thought to the human condition, once said, "The doctor of the future will give no medicine, but will interest his patients in the care of the human frame, in diet, and in the cause and prevention of disease." That was in 1931. A nutritionist of the highest professional standing in our own time, Dr. Paavo Airola, has put the same matter more bluntly: "If doctors of today will not become the nutritionists of tomorrow, then the nutritionists of today will become the doctors of tomorrow." There is some evidence, unfortunately inconclusive, that younger doctors of medicine are beginning to get the message.

It is not, of course, in the direct province of visual-training optometrists to prescribe proper diet for their eye patients, and none of the new school practitioners does so in any formal way, to the best of our knowledge. Occasionally they may recommend a nutritional corrective. Yet it is surprising they do not do it more systematically, for they find increasing evidence that visual deficiencies in their patients are related to deficiencies elsewhere in the system, and that these are frequently the direct consequence of faulty nutritional patterns—constant overeating, too many drugs, too much tobacco and alcohol. Lack of exercise and lack of rest and relaxation are related causes of body/mind deficiencies. In all cases, a proper diet is an essential ingredient of a visual-training program, for while the primary aim of the training is to improve the patient's vision, improvement can be sustained only by a condition of general health and harmony throughout the body/mind system.

The authors of this book have a special interest in nutrition and the value of a good diet. Moreover, as a consequence of her own long bout with ill health, Ann Hoopes is a serious student of nutrition, believing that it was the single most important factor in counteracting the several systemic derangements that made her life a misery for half a dozen years. She is the chairman of a health-food store in Washington, called *Yes!*, and thus almost daily involved in the study of nutrition on a practical level. Against the background of this experience, we set down here our own views on proper diet for whatever benefit they may be to the reader. You will find they are not dramatically different from other sensible, balanced diets; indeed, we have found that all serious students of nutrition have come to essentially the same conclusions about what is best for high energy and super-health:

137

Basic Foods	Foods to Avoid
grain cereals (especially buckwheat)	caffeinated drinks (especially
rye bread	coffee)
skim milk (sparingly)	white bread
eggs (sparingly)	pies, cakes
honey	sugar and sugared foods
nuts and seeds (especially peanuts,	fried foods
almonds, sesame, sunflower and	red meat
pumpkin seeds)	
fresh vegetables	
fresh fruits	
fruit and vegetable juices	
plain yogurt	
fish	
chicken/turkey (sparingly)	
green salad with oil (2 large	
helpings daily)	
water (6 glasses daily)	

A high-protein diet has come to be regarded as the symbol of health and energy (as well as of American affluence), and it is an important factor in nutrition. Americans, alas, have a tendency to carry good things beyond the bounds of proportion, and there is now evidence that excess protein—meaning more than can be thoroughly assimilated—can be harmful.

Vegetables and fruits purchased at grocery stores should be washed thoroughly with soap to remove the chemical sprays used to protect them from insects. All fruits should be eaten raw, and most vegetables; if vegetables are cooked, it should be lightly in a steamer, for overcooked (boiled) vegetables lose most of their nutritional value. The lowly potato, particularly if baked and eaten with its skin, is an especially valuable food. Also, contrary to common belief, potatoes are no more fattening than other vegetables.

Refined white sugar is perhaps the worst possible of all

foods, and has been referred to by concerned scientists as the "white poison" and the "white plague" of the civilized world. It is bad because it is a fragmented, adulterated, and denatured substance. Sugarcane and sugar beets are natural foods, but white sugar made from them has been wholly stripped of all the nutritional value present in the original; as a result, it causes serious problems in the body's metabolism. Unfortunately, refined sugar is very hard to avoid in our civilization because nearly all mass-produced commercial foods—soft drinks, ice cream, bread, cookies, pies, cakes, canned foods, baby foods, and dry breakfast cereals—are loaded with it.

What can the individual do? He can try to structure his diet so that it is minimally dependent on commercially produced food, and he can lend his support to the increased production of natural food. One brief case history concerning an older woman will demonstrate both the hazards of poor diet and too many drugs, and the ways in which good diet can reinforce visual training to relieve stress and bring about an improved general performance.

Gertrude

Gertrude is a woman in her middle seventies who had progressively lost her health through a series of afflictions including colitis, cancer of the lower intestine, and an unusual blood problem that caused her to produce too many red corpuscles and required doctors to withdraw blood from her system several times each month. The various drugs given her to relieve pain or alleviate these conditions appeared to contribute to digestive irregularities. Her husband died in 1975 after a long illness that had required her to spend many hours at his bedside, day and night. As a consequence, she was exhausted and both emotionally and physically stressed.

In the fall of 1976 she suffered what appeared to be the final blow: her retinas began to hemorrhage, and thus quickly blocked out her central vision, leaving unimpaired only a thin slit of peripheral vision as her one remaining window on the world. By any objective measure she was legally blind, unable to read, sew, drive a car, and able to feed herself and do her housekeeping only with great difficulty. Her doctors sadly concluded there was nothing to be done. "They told me in effect that nature had to take its course."

Through Ann Hoopes, Gertrude went to see a reputable nutritionist, Dr. Francis Woidich, who found her in an extremely run-down condition and alive "only because you possess such an inherently sturdy constitution." Being strong, she had been entirely unconcerned about what she ate. He found her system almost entirely devoid of vitamin B. He urged her to withdraw gradually from the various drugs she was taking, and he put her on a strict diet of grain cereals, fresh fruits and vegetables, fruit and vegetable juices, supplemented by liver shots and a wide range of vitamins. He then sent her to a visual-training optometrist. After examining her eyes, the doctor concluded that her basic problem was stress, and that there was nothing seriously wrong with her eyes. He worked out a treatment of hot and cold compresses on the eyes, daily walks, and a series of simple eye exercises to be done at home.

Gertrude undertook the new diet, the walking, and the eye exercises with a zeal born of desperation and hope. Within ten days, her central vision began to clear enough so that she could see objects within three or four feet; after two weeks she could read the headlines of *The New York Times*. A month later she was able to read an entire book. Her daily walks, which she gradually extended to nearly two miles, became a source of great refreshment and relaxation, and helped both to strengthen her body and to clarify her visual perception. The new diet stabilized her digestion and, in conjunction with the liver and vitamin supplements, gave her new energy and a calmer nervous system. The eye exercises improved her eye muscles and the clarity of her vision. "It's really like a miracle," she told Ann Hoopes. "If only someone had told me years ago about these natural cures."

It should not be necessary to add to this brief commentary on diet that smoking, particularly cigarette smoking, is severely detrimental not only to your lungs but also to your entire nervous system and to tissues throughout your body; nor that alcohol is a poison (albeit in some forms a pleasant one) that should be used in greater moderation with every passing year. As we have previously noted, a number of visual-training patients have voluntarily given up cigarettes and alcohol as a result of their training. The stress in their eyes and bodies having been removed or reduced by the training, they no longer felt the need for these crutches.

The central point here is simply that if you are serious about improving your vision and the general efficiency of your whole body/mind system, you must be serious about the nutritional quality of the food and drink you put into that system.

Exercise

The essence of the new school method is to create movement —to change the patient's visual mode and thus, inexorably, his physical mode as well. The visual-training program thus involves some physical conditioning, especially activities like walking and swimming that serve to balance out the body and create a supple muscle tone. There are two specific reasons for this emphasis on moderate physical conditioning: one is to permit the patient to carry out the eye and body exercises in the program without undue fatigue, and they can be quite tiring if done conscientiously; the other is to permit him to take more or less in stride the changes in posture—the actual shifting of muscles and blood vessels, initially in the neck and upper back, but ultimately involving shifts in other parts of the body—that accompany and follow changes in the visual system.

The benefits to health of regular, vigorous exercise are by now well known. Appropriate exercise can increase the lung capacity up to eight or ten times, which means a larger and more efficient distribution of oxygen throughout the body. This not only improves muscle tone generally, but also increases the flow of oxygen and other nutrients to the brain cells. By strengthening both the muscle tone and the cardiovascular system, regular exercise provides a protective cushion against stress, fatigue, and the dangers of heart attack; it promotes good posture, slows down the aging process, and is an effective cure for a number of ailments, including tension headaches and minor allergies. It is a medical truth that exercise, by increasing the efficiency of the whole organism, *generates* energy.

The physical conditioning most relevant to visual training involves aerobic exercises to strengthen the cardiovascular system, and balancing exercises to improve body awareness, coordination, and timing. The most common and popular aerobics are jogging, cycling, walking, swimming, and skipping rope. Jogging is an excellent conditioner of heart, lungs, and legs, and also promotes weight control; while it is perhaps best for people under 50, it can bring benefits to reasonably fit persons of all ages. Cycling brings similar benefits with somewhat less exertion. Swimming is an ideal conditioner because it exercises all the muscles of the body without stress; moreover, it develops longer, smoother muscles than certain other sports, and it also helps to control weight. Calisthenics are a splendid means of developing added body strength and flexibility, but they do not have a direct aerobic effect unless performed rigorously at a rapid pace. Tennis is a splendid conditioning activity, good for developing a flexible, balanced, well-proportioned body, and excellent for weight control; moreover, the visual complexities of following a fast-moving tennis ball, judging the space/time relationships between ball and racquet, ball and opponent, ball and court, constitute very practical eye exercises.

Training optometrists place varying degrees of emphasis on physical conditioning generally and on the value of particular kinds of exercising. Dr. Shankman, for example, recognizes a direct correlation between physical condition and progress in visual improvement and body/mind coordination, but is inclined to let each patient decide how vigorous a regimen he wants or needs. Those patients who are younger or determined to achieve a level of super-health, or those whose visual condition is desperate, may elect a tough, demanding program of jogging and calisthenics every day; other Shankman patients, with lower aspirations or less serious visual problems, may content themselves with regular walking. Dr. Streff appears to be similarly permissive, and to feel that regular jogging is too strenuous for most patients.

Of the training optometrists we have observed, Dr. Francke appears to demand the most from his patients, often requiring them to run or walk four miles a day, sleep ten hours, and change their dietary habits for a period of several weeks or months before he will admit them to his training program. His principal reasons for this "tough" approach appear to be a desire to protect them against the sometimes severe discomforts of physical changes—the so-called transitions—and a desire to see them come as close as possible to achieving what he terms their "optimum visual performance." Dr. Francke's classroom and home training programs are also somewhat more intensive than those of other doctors.

Whatever their differences on physical conditioning, however, all visual-training optometrists appear to agree wholeheartedly that walking is the ideal exercise for improving vision and balancing out the body/mind system. They find it is superior to jogging, swimming, or calisthenics, although they prescribe and encourage all of these activities and other active sports as well. A combination is best, but walking, Dr. Francke says, is "the single most effective means of bringing the whole body into biological balance." For when you are walking, "you balance out by letting the vision take over and tell you what physical adjustments to make. Vision is the master control mechanism, and if you walk correctly— with a long easy stride, arms swinging freely, stomach sucked in, head held erect as though some invisible force were pulling you straight up into the sky, and eyes taking in as much space as possible—you will continually improve the scope and depth and clarity of your field of vision." Why is this so? Because, Dr. Francke says, "walking outdoors, where the volume of space is large and the texture of the scenery richly varied, facilitates visually directed and verified postural adjustments. You make gross adjustments of the shoulders, hips, hands, and feet; and these lead, via the eye-brain feed-back mechanism, to ever finer adjustments of the eyes and thus to a clearer view of the real world." In short, the master secret of good body/mind coordination is visual feedback from *self-produced* movement.

Ten

Do You Need Help?

AS ALL of the foregoing chapters have sought to show, the new school method of visual training is primarily concerned with vision, yet is also unavoidably concerned with the impact that good or poor eyesight has upon the whole range of muscular and mental functions. The new school practitioners have no desire to impinge upon other areas of science or medicine, and they strenuously resist attempts by some people to define the new visual training as a form of psychobiology. They insist, correctly, that visual training is basically an advanced form of physical training. At the same time, they cannot escape the clinically observed truth that the visual system is the dominant sensory system, the principal mechanism of control, the one that plays an apparently decisive role in organizing and coordinating all of the various functions of the organism, including the brain.

Dr. A. M. Skeffington once observed that "he who is unstable in his visual world is insecure in his ego." We have shown by reference to selected case histories that this is true, that persons with stressed or seriously deficient visual performance often lack self-confidence and steady nerves, and often manifest undesirable personality traits and patterns of behavior. We have also shown that visual training, by treating the body/mind system as an essential unity, can produce improvements extending beyond visual scope and acuity to posture, muscular coordination, energy, creative powers—and even to behavior and personality. Effective visual training has brought an end not only to blurred vision but also to menstrual cramps, hay fever, and acne; it has strengthened intellectual performance and creativity and has changed irritable, complaining personalities into calm, self-confident men and women who are willing to assume full responsibility for their own shortcomings.

These results are not easily understood or accepted by the current conventional wisdom in medicine. And, beyond a certain level of generality, they are not easily explainable even by the professional optometrists who practice visual training. No one knows precisely how and why some things happen. There is indeed a certain mystery at the heart of the process. The new school optometrists are engaged in a fascinating clinical process whose methods and conclusions are being continuously tested and refined by the basic, old-fashioned method of open-minded observation, but this is not a method currently fashionable in medicine or indeed in other disciplines. In an age of computers and programmed learning, we all have a tendency to assume that every aspect of life is fully explainable, or should be. We forget that most of today's "hard science" started a number of years ago as someone's clear-eyed observation or intuitive hunch. We fail to remember that every successful creative effort in the history of mankind succeeded because it defied and moved beyond the accepted boundaries of conventional wisdom.

With respect to visual training, however, there is no need for timidity in the face of conventional doubts. The new visual training exists and it works. It is apparent that it works because it is soundly grounded in basic truths about the nature of the human organism. We have no doubt at all that a very large number of people in our overstressed society could be relieved of endless headaches, backaches, chronic exhaustion, and a whole range of minor ailments and disorders (and even some serious ones) if they were willing and able to undertake a properly defined visual-training program; moreover, we are sure that such relief could be the springboard to more positive, energetic, and productive lives.

While visual training is not yet available widely enough to serve all those who need it, the number of serious and dedicated professional training optometrists is steadily growing, and we believe that time and the spreading awareness of its social usefulness will increase the public demand and thus lead to its wider availability. It is our earnest hope that this book will play a constructive part in this process.

We close by posing a series of questions, developed in collaboration with several training optometrists, that amount to a visual self-evaluation test aimed at helping you determine whether your own visual system is functioning efficiently. If you will consider each question with careful, critical reflection on your own personal situation, you should be able to gain a sense of whether you need visual training, either to correct a specific visual problem or to alleviate a more general discomforting condition elsewhere in your body that may be related to the way your eyes are functioning.

1. Do you have a hard time driving a car?
2. Does oncoming traffic sometimes appear to be on your side of the road?
3. Do you have a tendency to put on your brakes fifty or sixty feet before you come to a stop sign? And do you jam on the brakes at each stop?
4. Do you have any other problems of judging depth when you drive?
5. When you walk, does the horizon appear to move up and down?
6. When you see objects, are they really where they appear to be, or do you often misjudge their true position and sometimes bump into them?
7. Do you play tennis, basketball, volleyball, or any other games involving moving balls and players?
8. If you don't, have you ever asked yourself why you don't?
9. If you play games with moving balls, but in a rather clumsy or mediocre way, how do you analyze your shortcomings?
10. In tennis, for example, do you frequently hit the ball on the edge of the racquet or miss it completely?
11. In basketball or baseball, can you pass and catch the ball easily? Can you shoot baskets accurately, or catch a fly ball in center field?
12. How do you rate your eye-brain-hand coordination?
13. Are you disturbed by crowds in theaters, department stores, or shopping centers?
14. Do you avoid frequenting such places?
15. Do objects appear the same size to you at thirty inches and thirty feet?
16. Does it bother you to walk in the dark with your eyes closed?

17. Are you a slow reader?
18. Can you organize your visual and mental capacities to read and write effectively, or are you disappointed by your performance?
19. Can you accurately reproduce—by drawing or written explanation—what you have just seen?
20. Can you apply these same capacities to solving practical or theoretical problems without the use of pencil and paper? Are you satisfied with your efficiency?
21. If the situation permits or requires, can you read or study for three hours or longer without suffering eye-strain and excessive fatigue?
22. Do you experience any lag in seeing clearly when you shift your attention from the TV screen across the room to the book in your hand, or vice versa?
23. Does your stomach bother you after sustained use of your eyes?
24. Are you happy with your overall physical and mental performance? If you are unhappy about this, can you identify the causes, stresses, or blockages that may be responsible for your performing at below your capacity?

If, after pondering these questions, you conclude that visual training would help your situation, get in touch with a professional optometrist in your neighborhood or town. If he is not engaged in visual training, show him this book and ask him if he can recommend a training optometrist. If that does not prove satisfactory, then write to the Optometric Extension Program, Duncan, Oklahoma 73533, and ask them to recommend a qualified training professional located in your general vicinity.

A final word. The new visual training offers the prospect of extraordinary benefit to those who are motivated to undertake it. Total performance is the payoff. The only basic requirement is motivation, but, as Aldous Huxley has written, this is the rub for many people: "Visual reeducation demands from the pupil a certain amount of thought, time and trouble. But thought, time and trouble are precisely what the overwhelming majority of men and women are not prepared to give unless motivated by a passionate desire or an imperious need. Most of us who can get along more or less satisfactorily with the help of mechanical seeing aids will continue to do so, even when they know there exists a system of training which would make it possible for them not merely to palliate symptoms, but actually to get rid of the causes of visual defect."

There is no overriding reason why you should accept the passive stance of the majority on a matter of such surpassing importance to your personal well-being.

Glossary

Accommodation: The ability of the eye to focus at either near point or distance.

Acuity: The ability to see clearly and sharply. Near-point acuity is clear sight at short ranges; distance acuity is clear sight at longer ranges.

Anisometropia: The condition of a different refractive or "seeing" power in each eye.

Astigmatism: The eye's inability to achieve a clear focus on any point, owing to unequal refractive power as between the vertical and the horizontal; sometimes caused by a faulty curvature of the cornea.

Binocular fusion: The condition in which both eyes achieve an identical, mutually reinforcing focus on the same object.

Cyclotorsion: A condition in which one or both eyes break the binocular fusion and show a tendency to rotate, out of control.

Diopter: The unit of measure of lens power. A one diopter lens produces convergence at a distance of one meter. A two diopter lens produces convergence either at two meters or at one half a meter, depending on whether its lens is concave or convex.

Doubling glasses: Lens combinations, used for training purposes only, that prevent the eyes from seeing any object singly.

Duction (low): A measurement of poor accommodation and/ or poor convergence.

Esophoria: A condition of overconvergence at either near point or distance.

Esotropic: The tendency of one eye to turn inward toward the nose.

Horizontal prism: A lens used to correct a horizontal imbalance between the two eyes.

Hyperopia: The condition of farsightedness; an inability to achieve acuity at near point owing to a weakness of focusing power.

Minus lens: A concave lens that is used for nearsightedness.

Myopia: The condition of nearsightedness, the inability to achieve visual acuity beyond a few feet.

Ophthalmologist: A specialist in the pathology of the eye— e.g., glaucoma and cataracts.

Optometrist: A health professional who performs eye examinations to determine the presence of visual, muscular, or neurological abnormalities and prescribes lenses, other optical aids, or therapy to achieve maximum vision. Optometrists are also trained to recognize disease conditions of the eye and ocular manifestations of other diseases, and to refer patients with these conditions to the appropriate medical doctor.

Orthomolecular psychiatrist: A psychiatrist who uses vitamins, chemical testing, and physical testing to assist his diagnosis and treatment.

Pediatrician: A specialist in child care.

Peripheral vision: That which is seen all around the central field of vision; good peripheral vision is essential for defining accurate spatial relationships.

Plus lens: A convex lens that is used for farsightedness.

Glossary

Postural set: The bodily position or carriage resulting from the interplay of the visual system and the muscular structure.

Postural warp: The sum of the postural deviations caused by the body's effort to compensate for visual deficiencies.

Retinoscope: An instrument that records various levels of light intensity in the eyes when the organism confronts a variety of situations.

Rotating prisms: Lenses, used for training only, that can be rotated within their frames to vary the power and direction of the lens.

Strabismus: The condition of being cross-eyed.

20/20 sight: A measurement of the Snellen rating system indicating that the eyes can distinguish and discriminate letters of a certain size at a distance of 20 feet.

Vertical phoria: The tendency of one eye to look upward rather than to project horizontally in parallel with the other eye.

Vertical prism: A lens used to correct a vertical imbalance between the two eyes.

Vision: The faculty of sight.

Notes

Introduction

page xiv: "it shows people . . ."
Conversation with John Streff, June 8, 1978.

Chapter 1

pages 4–5: . . . a remarkable man . . . reexamining his own positions.
Arthur Hoare, "The Skeffington Saga. Part 1 (Skeffington—The Man),"
Optometric World, May 1966.

page 6: "an affront and insult . . ."
Education, Vol. 79, No. 2 (October 1958).

pages 9–10: Most ophthalmologists, . . . Huxley wrote . . . "the force of
habit and authority that we do all accept it."
Aldous Huxley, *The Art of Seeing* (1942; published in paperback by
Montana Books, Inc., 1975), pp. 1–4.

page 10: . . . several significant scientific developments . . .
Charles Murgach, "Tenets of Functional Optometry," *Review of Optometry,* Vol. 113, June–July 1976.

page 12: . . . compensatory, remedial and developmental.
Louis Bates Ames, Clyde Gillespie, and John Streff, *Stop School Failure*
(New York: Harper & Row, 1972), pp. 129–34.

Chapter 3

page 27: Together . . . "dynamic balance"
Charles Sherrington, *The Integrative Actions of the Nervous System*
(New Haven: Yale University Press, 1947), p. 50.

Notes

page 27: . . . a primary function of the visual system . . .
Darrell Boyd Harmon, *A Dynamic Theory of Vision,* monograph (1948).

page 27: The reverse is also true.
Ibid.

pages 33–34: "the level of efficiency . . ."
Conversation with Dr. Amiel Francke, 1976.

page 34: Vision is the "lead system."
Conversation with Dr. John Streff, June 7, 1978.

page 36: Dr. Leonard Cohen . . .
Leonard Cohen, "Mechanisms of Perception: Their Development and Function," paper prepared for the Perceptual-Motor Symposium, May 8–10, 1968, Washington, D.C.

page 38: "plastic seeing mechanism"
Arnold Gesell, *Vision: Its Development in Infant and Child* (New York: Harper & Bros., 1949), p. 33.

pages 38–39: This principle . . . that balanced development . . .
Ibid., pp. 34–35.

page 39: Two factors were crucial . . .
Ibid., p. 39.

page 40: "new conquests in the sphere of vision"
Ibid., p. 41.

Chapter 4

page 42: "human action system . . . the retina and the brain."
Gesell, *Vision,* p. 13.

page 42: ". . . most direct corridor . . . in vision."
Ibid., p. 172.

pages 42–43: Darrell Boyd Harmon . . . intellectual experience.
Harmon, *A Dynamic Theory of Vision.*

page 43: Dr. John Streff has explained . . .
Conversation with Dr. John Streff, June 8, 1978.

page 43: . . . "a kind of meeting ground . . ."
Gesell, *Vision,* p. 168.

Notes

page 44: Moreover, the building of the . . . space world . . . has gone before."
D. O. Hebb, *The Organization of Behavior* (New York: John Wiley & Sons, 1949), p. 109.

pages 44–45: Dr. Streff explains. . . . Vision is thus a conditioned response
Conversation with Dr. John Streff, June 8, 1978.

page 45: "We see what we're set to see . . ."
Conversation with Dr. Lawrence W. Macdonald, January 1978.

page 46: "no one-to-one relationship . . ."
Conversation with Dr. Amiel Francke, 1977.

page 55: "The net effect . . . development in girls."
Ames *et al., Stop School Failure,* pp. 143–44.

pages 55–56: According to Dr. John Streff . . .
Conversation with Dr. John Streff, June 8, 1978.

page 56: Environment and work intensity . . .
Ames *et al., Stop School Failure,* p. 144.

pages 56–58: Dr. Amiel Francke . . .
Amiel Francke and William K. Carr, "Culture and the Development of Vision," *Journal of American Optometry,* January 1976.

pages 61–62: Dr. Albert Shankman . . .
Conversation with Dr. Albert Shankman, January 1978.

page 62: Given the pervasive interaction . . . perceptions by the brain.
K. S. Lashley, *The Problems of Serial Order* (New York: John Wiley & Sons, 1951), p. 128.

page 62: As a viewing person . . . your cumulative experience.
Gesell, *Vision,* p. 174.

page 67: . . . computor flow-chart analogy . . .
Lawrence W. Macdonald, "Optometric Regimens: A Syndrome Approach," paper published by the Optometric Extension Program, 1977.

Chapter 5

page 69: "struggle . . . parts within the whole."
Hans Selye, *The Stress of Life* (New York: McGraw-Hill Book Company, 1976), p. 12.

page 70: "Physiologic aging . . . never wastefully for worthless efforts."
Ibid., p. 428.

page 71: . . . a net depletion
Ibid., p. 429.

page 71: "We invariably die . . . weakest vital link"
Ibid., p. 431.

page 71: "the manifest features"
Ibid., p. 435.

page 72: "The great art . . . foresaw for us."
Ibid., p. 419.

page 72: "The human body . . . wears evenly."
Ibid., p. 433.

page 73: A number of studies . . . stimuli as ever.
Arnold Friedhoffer and Manfred Warren, *The Effect of Near Point Visual Demands upon the Central Visual Field,* monograph (1970).

page 73: But, as Dr. Streff has noted . . .
Conversation with Dr. John Streff, June 8, 1978.

page 74: Dr. Shankman believes . . .
Conversation with Dr. Albert Shankman, August 1978.

page 74: Other studies . . . comprehension and personality.
Virginia Shipman, "The Restriction of the Perceptual Field under Stress," paper presented to the Eastern Psychological Association, January 1954.

pages 83–84: "vision is . . . range of involuntary functions."
Talk with Dr. John Streff, June 8, 1978.

Chapter 6

page 86: "a self-monitoring . . . of the patient."
Macdonald, "Optometric Regimens."

page 88: "getting patients . . . mismatches."
Lawrence W. Macdonald, "Implications of Critical Empathy, Primal Scream and Identity Crisis in Optometric Visual Therapy," *Journal of the American Optometric Association,* October 1972.

pages 90–91: Dr. Streff compares . . . around him.
Ames, *et al., Stop School Failure,* p. 138.

page 92: Dr. Shankman's patients . . . coordination and control.
Conversation with Dr. Albert Shankman, August 1978.

page 92: A number of his training patients . . . improved, too.
Ibid.

page 93: Dr. Macdonald believes . . . body posture.
Macdonald, "Implications of Critical Empathy . . ."

page 94: Self-awareness forces . . . feedback mechanism.
Ibid.

page 100: Dr. Francke made an assessment . . .
Conversation with Dr. Amiel Francke, August 1977.

Chapter 7

page 105: as Dr. Shankman expressed it . . .
Talk with Dr. Albert Shankman, January 1978.

page 106: Dr. Macdonald has said plainly . . .
Macdonald, "Optometric Regimens."

page 107: "these are not sequential . . . for everyone."
Conversation with Dr. Amiel Francke, 1976.

page 107: "it is amazing . . . with a willing patient."
Macdonald, "Optometric Regimens."

page 107: "When the program . . . practicing."
Ibid.

page 112: Herman A. Witkin has described . . .
Herman A. Witkin, "The Perception of the Upright," *Scientific Americans,* February 1959.

pages 115–16: ask yourself the following questions:
Dr. Amiel Francke, "Introduction to Optometric Visual Training," paper published by Optometric Extension Program, 1974.

Chapter 8

page 129: what Dr. Streff calls . . . beyond the word.
Talk with Dr. John Streff, June 8, 1978.

pages 130–31: Dr. Streff emphasizes . . . "constriction of myopia."
Ibid.

Chapter 9

page 136: Thomas A. Edison . . .
Quoted in preface to *Reams Diet Booklet* (GMS Enterprises, 1977).

page 136: "If doctors of today . . ."
Paavo Airola, *How to Get Well* (Phoenix, Ariz.: Health Plus Publishers, 1974), p. 24.

pages 138–39: Refined white sugar . . . body's metabolism.
Paavo Airola, *Hypoglycemia: A Better Approach* (Phoenix, Ariz.: Health Plus Publishers, 1977), p. 56.

pages 144–45: "the single most effective means . . . view of the real world."
Talk with Dr. Amiel Francke, 1977.

Chapter 10

page 151: "Visual reeducation . . . visual defect."
Huxley, *The Art of Seeing,* p. 11.

Index

163

Index

Ann M. Hoopes was born in Cleveland, Ohio, in 1933, and grew up in Wilmette, Illinois, and Southport, Connecticut. She was educated at Wellesley College and the University of Bridgeport. She is an accomplished pianist, a member of the National Symphony Board, and chairman of Yes!, a health food store and bookstore in Washington.

Townsend Hoopes was born in Duluth, Minnesota, in 1922 and was educated at Andover and Yale University. He served as a Marine Corps officer in World War II. From 1965 through 1968 he held several policy positions in the Defense Department, including Undersecretary of the Air Force. His book on Vietnam, *The Limits of Intervention,* won the Overseas Writers Prize for the best book on foreign affairs in 1969. His 1973 biography, *The Devil and John Foster Dulles,* won a Bancroft History Prize. He is now president of the Association of American Publishers.

The text of this book was set on the Linotype in a type face called Baskerville. The face is a facsimile reproduction of types cast from molds made for John Baskerville (1706–75) from his designs. The punches for the revived Linotype Baskerville were cut under the supervision of the English printer George W. Jones.

John Baskerville's original face was one of the fore-runners of the type style known as "modern face" to printers—a "modern" of the period A.D. 1800.